I MUST
DECREASE

I MUST DECREASE

Inspiration & Encouragement for Dieters

Janice Thompson

BARBOUR
PUBLISHING

Cover image © th**inkpen** DESIGN

The author is represented by The Knight Agency, Inc.

Published by Barbour Publishing, Inc., P.O. Box 719, Uhrichsville, Ohio 44683, www.barbourbooks.com

Our mission is to publish and distribute inspirational products offering exceptional value and biblical encouragement to the masses.

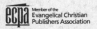

Member of the
Evangelical Christian
Publishers Association

Printed in the United States of America
5 4 3 2

This book is dedicated to Martha Rogers, a "lightweight" bundle of energy who always motivates me to do the right thing, and to the ladies of Lighter Writers:

You have truly been the wind beneath these tubby wings. I can't thank you enough.

Foreword

As an eating disorder specialist for more than twenty years, I take special joy in teaming with individuals to accomplish their health and weight goals. Sometimes, people approach weight loss in weariness and frustration. For this reason, unique approaches that "color outside the lines" are especially appealing. You'll find that *I Must Decrease* is refreshing, renewing, and revitalizing!

Here's how to best maximize this delightful, biblically sound resource: Read it. Laugh! Read it again. Laugh again! Allow your perspective to change. Use this book to renew your thinking. Connect with the healing humor in these pages. Integrate the wisdom into lifelong change for good. Celebrate fresh victories and you'll find yourself farther down the road to success.

Let Janice Thompson be your friend. She knows the pain, the bumps in the road. She'll be with you as you move beyond the deep valleys. Let her be your guide to the heights of joy. Like Janice, keep believing in your God-directed destiny. Follow the action steps and find your way to success! Proverbs 15:13 tells us that "a happy heart makes the face cheerful, but heartache crushes the spirit." *I Must Decrease* will allow you to maneuver around the heartache and have a happy heart.

Blessings!

GREGORY L. JANTZ, PH.D., C.E.D.S.
Author of *Hope, Help, and Healing for Eating Disorders*

Author's Note

For most of my life, I've known and loved the Lord and tried to live according to the precepts in His Word. For most of my life, I've struggled with a weight problem, pretending it didn't exist. It wasn't until a few years ago that I began to see how those two things were intricately tied together. After all, God entrusted this vessel to me, but I wasn't doing a very good job caring for it. With four daughters to raise, a husband to care for, classes to teach, and books to write, who had time to worry about dieting?

Not me. And obviously not a lot of others in the church either. All I had to do was look down the church pew to find many folks in the same boat. So we were a little tubby. Who cared? We went out to lunch together after church on Sundays. We planned church socials together. None of my fellow believers seemed to care that my weight was ballooning, any more than I worried about their expanding waistlines. I felt their love and I'm sure they felt mine.

In 2002, I felt the Lord's nudging and I knew I couldn't ignore His voice any longer. As a Christian drama team director who yearned to travel, I had no doubt that God would eventually take me across the globe to spread the gospel message. However, with 275 pounds on a 5 foot 2 inch frame, I had a "small" problem. Just fitting comfortably into the airplane seat could prove to be my undoing. How in the world could I climb mountains, scale heights, and reach the lost?

Should I start a diet? Again? Every time I thought about it, I cringed. I'd been down that road several times already and had never finished well. No, dieting was not for me, and if anyone asked why, I had plenty of excuses, including my Top Ten list:

1. God loves me just the way I am.
    True, but He loves me too much to leave me that way.

2. My husband loves me just the way I am.
   He'd better! Real love sees beyond all the flaws.

3. I'm happy with myself.
   Happy/content/unwilling to change. . .it's all relative, right?

4. I come from a long line of overweight people.
   Hmm. . .I wonder how my children and grandchildren will feel about that?

5. Fat people don't wrinkle.
   This is very important to a woman in her forties. Of course, I do want to live to see my fifties, sixties, and beyond. . .

6. My children use me as a pillow.
   Not that I necessarily want to be compared to a pillow. . .

7. Fat people are happy people.
   Visions of a jolly Santa Claus dance before my eyes.

8. I have no willpower.
   Oops! I forgot this was God's battle, not mine!

9. I don't own a scale.
   Easily remedied. . .

10. I dieted before and gained all the weight back. I can't do this again. I just can't.
    Ah. Finally something logical.

As a result of these and other excuses, I found myself in the worst shape of my life. Besides the obvious struggles of a severely overweight person, I battled sleep apnea, waking with a migraine nearly every morning, caused by lack of oxygen. I was borderline diabetic. My cholesterol was elevated and my energy level was so low I could barely function. Getting out of bed was a challenge, and doing basic things—like housework—was difficult. It was beyond time for a change and I could no longer ignore the Lord's nudging.

Breaking the Cycle

How does one go about changing a forty-three-year habit? What is the key? Ironically, I found it to be so simple that it almost scared me. The answer lies in one word: *Decide.*

That's it?

That's it. It's so uncomplicated, really. It's the same principle you use every day of your life in other ways. How did you know which college to attend? You decided. How did you know which house to buy? You decided. How did you know which job to take? You decided. How did you know whether or not to follow the Lord? You decided.

The decision to lose weight is half the battle. Once the decision is made, the mind prepares the body to obey. The human spirit aligns itself with the Spirit of God, and the race begins. In all honesty, weight loss is not as difficult as we've made it out to be. We make it harder by placing unrealistic expectations on ourselves.

On January 16, 2002, I decided to lose weight. Every word in this book comes as a direct result of that decision. I pray the following pages will motivate and inspire you to come to a decision of your own. May God bless you on your journey.

JANICE THOMPSON

He must increase,
but I must decrease.

JOHN 3:30 NKJV

Preface: Preparing for the Race

At what point does the out-of-shape believer look in the mirror and say, "I should probably do something about this body of mine?" For some, the desire to "look better" kicks in when they enter their teens, a time of social competitiveness. For others, the need to "get healthy" seems more practical in their middle years, when they've come to the understanding that God expects them to care for the vessel He's entrusted to them. Many don't decide to do anything about their expanding waistlines until they're in their golden years. Some people merely gaze in the mirror with defeated looks on their faces and say, "I'd love to look better. I'd love to feel better. But I just don't think I can do it. I can't stand the idea of going on another diet."

It is for all of these people that this book has been written.

Diet is an ugly word. As soon as people hear it, they start getting nervous. "What will I have to give up? How long will I have to do without? What will I be asked to sacrifice today?" As soon as the word *sacrifice* enters the picture, their willpower fades. They feel defeated before they even begin. Panicked, they hit the bookstores, looking for answers.

And answers abound. Books on dieting are a dime a dozen. They tell you what to eat and—more frustrating—what not to eat. They tell you what to do and what not to do. They encourage you to look to yourself for the answers and to dig deep to find the willpower necessary to stick with whatever plan they present. In short, they claim to present the answer to your problem. However, there is only one answer to the world's dieting dilemma and it will never be found in a book. It is found in the person of Jesus Christ—our ultimate example of how to live a truly excellent life.

This is not a book about dieting. It is not a how-to manual. It advocates no particular plan and makes no promises, except those found in scripture. This sometimes humorous, sometimes serious devotional was written simply to bring encouragement to people who are interested in eating right and getting into shape. Whether you're thinking about losing weight, well along the way to your goal, or struggling mightily with a diet, you will find hope in the following pages.

This book is also a glimpse into the spiritual side of the willpower issue, and it offers serious, scriptural answers. I firmly believe that the quest to lose weight and get healthy can be a life-or-death struggle for Christians. There's nothing funny about the daily battle between right and wrong, good and evil. Is there any greater defeat than thinking you can't change? Perhaps one: thinking that you don't need to change. How refreshing, how enlightening, to discover that the power to change lies in the hand of the very One who created you! The battle is not yours, my friend. It never was.

Remember the story of David facing the mighty giant, Goliath? With those five smooth stones in his hand, young David began to boast in the Lord—before he even threw the first stone. Imagine how bold he must have appeared to those around him. You can be just as bold as you face the giants of gluttony and food addiction. With the Lord on your side, they will not defeat you. With the Lord on your side (and He is, you know), you can overcome.

But how? Where do you begin? Perhaps you're like I was, facing many, many years of neglect. Maybe you just want to drop a few pounds or maintain your current weight. Regardless of your goal, I have discovered some things that could be of interest to you.

The weight-loss journey seems to move in phases. The first leg is devoted to "getting started" or "gearing up." Motivation kicks in and—like a horse out of the gate—you begin to run. Sometimes a little too fast. That why the first section of this book has been titled "Off to the Races." How you approach the first part of the journey is essential to finishing well.

The second phase can prove to be a little more frustrating. Your weight plateaus, your patience wears thin, and you feel like throwing in the towel. This is often the point at which many people drop out of the race. I've titled the second section "Rounding the Turn," because this phase often forces us to remove our hands from the controls.

Finally, you pick up speed and move toward your goal. Just as you're approaching the finish line, you come to a startling realization: The race doesn't end here. You have to circle the track again. And again. The truth sinks in: Eating right is a forever thing. But you can do it. After all, look how far you've come! With this in mind, the last section of the book is titled "The Final Stretch." Here you will learn to embrace the positive lifestyle changes you've made—for the rest of your life.

Devotions in each section are divided into twelve categories:

Tickler: A humorous quote to tickle your funny bone

Tidbit: A "Did You Know?" feature, offering tidbits of information from multiple sources

Trap: Common misconceptions and/or food traps we often fall into

Trick: Tricks of the trade to help you stick with your plan

Treat: Clever snack and food ideas for healthy eaters

Testimony: Personal testimony from people (including some prominent personalities) who have faced the weight-loss challenge and won

Treasure: Daily scripture reference

Thought for the Day: Devotional thought for the day, based on the daily scripture verse

Turning Your Focus: A variety of ways you can reach out to help others

Trusting God: A brief prayer to help you admit your need for God's help

Today's Food Choices: A place to record your daily food choices

Thoughts on Paper (Daily Journal Entry): It helps to take the time to jot down personal things that happen each day, whether those things are good or bad. This is the place to list the things that God is doing in your life and to write down life lessons you learn along the way. Whenever you get discouraged, you can go back and read your notes.

Wherever you are in your weight-loss journey, be assured of one thing: The Lord loves you just as you are today. If you never lose a pound, He will continue to adore you. However, your merciful Father loves you enough to motivate you to care for the vessel you've been given. With that in mind, let's take a look at some humorous and inspirational thoughts to help you as you contemplate getting into shape and eating right.

Note: Always consult your doctor before beginning a dieting program. You may want to share the information in this book with him or her, as well.

All references to sugar should be taken in context and do not apply to diabetics. Always follow your personal doctor's instruction.

OFF TO THE RACES

> "A horse gallops with his lungs,
>   Perseveres with his heart,
>   and wins with his character."[1]
>
> TESIO

The horses are led to the gate against their will. Poking and prodding urge them into place, but they fight it every step of the way. Once inside, there's no turning back. They stand with bated breath, pawing at the ground and kicking against the closed metal doors that block their escape. A few soothing words from their riders and the animals seem to relax. Then, suddenly, they come alive. Nostrils flare and their breath comes more evenly. They set their sights on the course ahead and press the gate in anticipation. Everything within them yearns for the signal—the starting bell.

Finally! The gate flings open and the track announcer intones, "They're off and running!" The horses gallop like maniacs, full of vigor and strength. The crowd roars. Encouragement is at an all-time high. Their eyes are on the goal, the prize that lies ahead.

In many ways, the weight-loss journey is like a horse race. We may come to it after many years of fighting and kicking, but finally we decide: "This time. . .this time I'm going to do it." With a little urging from the Lord, we begin to prepare ourselves. We focus on the goal. We gather a crowd of encouragers around us. (They will be vital to our success.) When the big day comes, we enter the race with expectation and a surprising amount of zeal. We are invincible. Nothing can stop us. Or can it?

Tickler

A diet is when you have to go to some length to change your width.
Anonymous

Dieting Isn't for Me

Tickler
I'm in shape. Round is a shape, isn't it?
Author Unknown

Tidbit
Did You Know?

The word *diet* probably brings to mind meals of lettuce and cottage cheese. By definition, *diet* refers to what a person eats or drinks during the course of a day. A diet that limits portions to a very small size or that excludes certain foods entirely to promote weight loss may not be effective over the long term.[2]

> ### Trap
>
> Eating without thinking.
>
> Perhaps there is no bigger trap for the would-be healthy eater than simply not paying attention to what you eat. How often do we reach for something "just because"? We need to pay careful attention to everything we put in our mouths. Just this one act alone can make a difference in the size of our waistline.

Trick
Remove the word *diet* from your vocabulary and replace it with a term like *healthy eating*.

Testimony

I have struggled with weight issues for as long as I can remember. In my late twenties, I threw dieting out the window after gaining and losing nearly one hundred pounds. To be perfectly honest, I stopped caring about myself at some point along the way, but I didn't acknowledge it. I tried to pretend that my excess weight was no big deal. But inside I knew the truth. The problem was that I had tried the dieting route before, with immediate success—followed by swift failure. How could I accomplish the weight loss I desired without traditional dieting? With the Lord's help and guidance, I began to implement a simple plan. I cut back on food and I increased my exercise. Sounds easy, right? It wasn't always. But over a thirteen-month period, I dropped 110 pounds. I'll never "diet" again, but I will thank the Lord every day for teaching me healthy eating habits.

Janice Thompson

Treasure

"I do believe; help me overcome my unbelief!"
MARK 9:24

Thought for the Day

Why diet? My body has made it this far, so why bother? Wrestling with guilt and anxiety has never sounded like much fun, and dieting causes both, right? Why would I want to do that to myself? I've finally learned to love myself just the way I am. Why change now?

Truthfully, dieting isn't fun. Those who have dieted multiple times only to face failure at the end of their journey know all too well the price that dieters pay. Look up! There is good news. Dieting is not for you. It's not for anyone, in fact. Anything that causes despair, doubt, or confusion is not for believers. However, the Lord still expects us to do something about those excess pounds we've been carrying around. He loves us so much, and He wants the very best for His children. That's one of the reasons why He reminds us in his Word that our body is a temple—not just for His benefit as the Creator of that temple, but for our own benefit, as well.

················(Turning Your Focus)··············

Think of a friend who struggles with self-esteem issues.
Write him or her a card of encouragement today.

Trusting God

Lord, I have to admit I'm completely helpless when it comes to my eating habits. I need Your intervention. I need Your guidance and wisdom with every food choice, large or small. Help me place my trust in You, Lord—and give me the courage to make some changes in my life. Amen.

Today's Food Choices
(List all the foods you've eaten today)

_____

_____

_____

_____

Thoughts on Paper (Daily Journal Entry)

_____

_____

_____

_____

_____

_____

_____

_____

_____

_____

_____

_____

_____

_____

_____

_____

He Loves Me,
He Loves Me Not

Tickler

God loves us the way we are but
He loves us too much to leave us that way.
Leighton Ford

Tidbit

Did You Know?

You can rest secure in the love of the Lord. No matter what you do (or don't do), it won't affect His love for you.

⸱⸱⸱⸱⸱⸱⸱⸱⸱⸱⸱⸱⸱⸱⸱⸱(Trap)⸱⸱⸱⸱⸱⸱⸱⸱⸱⸱⸱⸱⸱

Pacifying ourselves with food.

We often reach for food when we should reach for the Word or cry out to the Lord in prayer. Learning to recognize these times is half the battle.

Trick

Write down a scripture from God's Word that confirms His love for you. Commit it to memory.

Testimony

I hate being overweight. I don't feel like this on the inside. I can't see the extra pounds and inches that make me try not to think about the eyes of others on me, that force me to shop in the "Plus" department away from my other friends who are more "normal" in size. Thank God for grace! He can see through this mess I've made of my body, and I know He'll honor my resolve to do better. He already has.

Lynette Sowell

Treasure

The Lord does not look at the things man looks at.
Man looks at the outward appearance,
but the Lord looks at the heart.
1 SAMUEL 16:7

Thought for the Day

People often decide that God loves or doesn't love them based on their behavior or appearance. Human beings love conditionally—and, in many cases, those who struggle with weight issues bear the brunt of teasing, ostracizing, or other displays of love loss. But God loves unconditionally. He looks at your heart, not your physical body. Of course, he cares about your health—but whether or not you "live by the dieting rules" doesn't affect His love for you. God wants to give you His best. This includes great health—both internally and externally. He wants you to be healthy spiritually, but He also wants to provide for you psychologically and emotionally. This is the gift of a loving God. He doesn't change.

Show God's love by offering to
clean the home of someone who's unable.

Trusting God

Father, I thank You that Your love is not conditional. Thank You for loving me in spite of my flaws. Teach me to rest in Your love and to walk confidently through each day as a result. Show me how to love others unconditionally, and give me strength for this journey, I pray. Amen.

Today's Food Choices
(List all the foods you've eaten today)

_____

_____

_____

_____

Thoughts on Paper (Daily Journal Entry)

_____

_____

_____

_____

_____

_____

_____

Oh, the Unfairness of It All

Tickler
The leading cause of death among fashion models is falling through street grates.
Dave Barry

Tidbit
Did You Know?

The average American woman is 5 feet 4 inches tall and weighs 140 pounds.

The average American female model is 5 feet 11 inches tall and weighs 117 pounds.

Most female fashion models are thinner than 98 percent of American women.[4]

(Trap)

Lack of balance.

We eat too much, then eat too little to make up for it. We diet all week and splurge on the weekend. The best way to handle small temptations is with small rewards. The key to success is to keep everything in balance.

Trick

Create your own runway. Start walking today—not for the roar of the crowd, but for your own health and enjoyment.

Treat

Do you think models eat like rabbits? Try a little rabbit food of your own. Combine granola with craisins (dried cranberries), raisins, or other dried fruit. Divide into ⅓-cup portions and place in resealable bags for a quick, sweet treat that's low in calories but high in fiber. Whenever the munchies attack, nibble away!

Testimony

Before sending a picture to my sister, I cut myself out. I had let my weight problem get out of control. God began to work on me through my doctor and the gentle voice of His Spirit within. My cholesterol level kept elevating even though I was taking medication for it. When I asked the doctor to increase it, he said, "No, not unless you lose weight. It wouldn't do any good." I realized I was not being a good witness to the ladies I was teaching in Bible study by not practicing self-control or taking care of God's temple, my body. The Spirit of the Lord led me to a weight-loss program and I successfully lost forty-three pounds through walking in the Spirit and practicing self-control.

Charlotte Holt

Treasure

Each one should test his own actions.
Then he can take pride in himself,
without comparing himself to somebody else,
for each one should carry his own load.
GALATIANS 6:4–5

Thought for the Day

Some things just don't seem fair, do they? Your friend eats a cheese-burger, fries, and a milkshake and stays trim. You eat a banana and gain three pounds. Who can explain it? Instead of giving up when these things occur, we need to learn to take our eyes off of others and focus only on the vessel the Lord has given us. Also, we need to deal with our insecurities and stop comparing ourselves to those around us, which often leads only to envy or other problems. Finally, we need to learn to trust God. How simple this sounds, and yet how difficult it is to do at times. Rest assured, the Lord is in control. He's got big plans for you (pardon the pun). He wants to use you in mighty ways and needs you to be in good shape to accomplish that. He's not comparing you to others, and neither should you.

$$\boxed{\text{Turning Your Focus}}$$

Visit with an elderly friend or neighbor.

Trusting God

Lord, today I start by asking You to forgive me for my jealousies and in-securities. Keep my eyes focused on You and not on others, Father. Help me not to worry about what others look like, or to compare myself to them. Thank You for placing value in me. Now give me the strength I need to become all You desire me to be. In Jesus' name. Amen.

Today's Food Choices

(List all the foods you've eaten today)

_____

_____

_____

_____

Thoughts on Paper (Daily Journal Entry)

Excuses, Excuses

Tickler

I've been on a constant diet for the last two decades.
I've lost a total of 789 pounds. By all accounts,
I should be hanging from a charm bracelet.
Erma Bombeck

Tidbit

Did You Know?

3,500 calories = one pound

Trap

Rewarding ourselves with food.

When we do well at work, we "go out with the girls" to celebrate over a high-calorie, high-fat lunch. When we get a promotion, we celebrate with cake or other sweets. It's time to stop rewarding ourselves with food and start rewarding ourselves with encouraging thoughts and words.

Trick

Tell someone about your decision to get healthy, but don't proclaim it to the masses. Making a "big deal" could inadvertently shift too much focus in your direction.

Testimony

We called my grandmother "Bubbie" Solomon. She was told by her doctor to adhere strictly to a newly prescribed diet. Aware of this, my dad observed her cooking a normal dinner (fried potato pancakes, cherry dumplings, boiled beef flank with onions, and kasha [buckwheat groats] with bow tie noodles in garlic sauce). He said, "Mom, what about the diet?" Bubbie Solomon replied, "First I eat supper, then I eat the diet."

Michael Solomon

Treasure

"Come now, let us reason together," says the LORD.
"Though your sins are like scarlet, they shall be as white as snow;
though they are red as crimson, they shall be like wool."
ISAIAH 1:18

Thought for the Day

We're all loaded with excuses about our weight, aren't we? We blame our extra pounds on genetics or on our mother's poor cooking habits. We blame our hectic rush-about schedules and lack of time for proper exercise. Though there may be some validity to these claims, we are still in charge of our own eating and exercising habits. Time restraints aside, there are few excuses for not taking a more positive approach to our bodies.

(Turning Your Focus)

If your parents are still living, write a memory of
a special time you had as a child and send it to them.

Trusting God

Lord, I have to admit that I've been full of excuses. Please forgive
me for not taking action sooner. Help me to see clearly past the fog
of impossibilities. Give me hope, Lord. Thank You for giving me the
courage to change. Amen.

Today's Food Choices

(List all the foods you've eaten today)

_____

_____

_____

_____

Thoughts on Paper (Daily Journal Entry)

_____

_____

_____

_____

_____

_____

_____

What's Eating You?

Tickler
Gluttony is an emotional escape, a sign something is eating us.
Peter De Vries

Tidbit
Did You Know?

To determine your Body Mass Index (BMI) using pounds and inches, multiply your weight in pounds by 704.5, then divide the result by your height in inches, and divide that result by your height in inches a second time.[5]

Trap

Quick fix snacks, such as candy bars.

It might be easier to reach for a candy bar rather than a healthy snack, but in the long run we will reap the rewards of our choices. We have trained ourselves to reach for certain things when we're bugged, and we need to be untrained. Also, we tend to create habits that are very difficult to undo. Next time you need a "quick fix," reach for a piece of fruit or something healthy to take the edge off.

Trick
Find out what's eating you. If you begin a diet but never solve your underlying problems, the weight won't stay off for very long.[6]

Testimony

My journey through life has been made especially difficult because of my issues with food. I never remember having a normal relationship with food, never knew what it meant to use food as fuel, never got the concept of "eat when you're hungry and stop when you're finished." All foreign concepts to me. My nickname (lovingly given to me by three older siblings) was "Piglet." They also called me "Two-bowls" in reference to how much cereal I would eat in the morning. Eating too much defined who I was in the family. I hated it. I hated myself for being this way but felt powerless to change.

Mary Hanlon

Treasure

For our struggle is not against flesh and blood,
but against the rulers, against the authorities,
against the powers of this dark world
and against the spiritual forces of evil in the heavenly realms.
EPHESIANS 6:12

Thought for the Day

Overeating is often caused by insecurity. We eat to hide what we're really thinking or feeling. How many times have you reached for a cookie or piece of cake to pacify yourself when hurt? Do you run to sweets when you're feeling particularly blue? If so, you might be an emotional eater. Remember, our struggles aren't against flesh and blood; neither are the answers to our struggles in the realm of flesh and blood. We can't combat spiritual forces with a pastry or a cream puff. If we were to be honest with ourselves, we'd have to admit that, more often than not, we try to solve our emotional dilemmas by eating them away. This type of behavior is not just bad for us, it is sinful. It causes us to reach out to "something" instead of "Someone." In moments of crisis, we must learn to bypass the chocolate chip cookies and reach out to Jesus instead.

Turning Your Focus

Tell a Sunday school teacher or pastor
what a great job he or she is doing.

Trusting God

Lord, I have to acknowledge that I haven't always come to You with my problems. Sometimes I've turned to other things, including food. Help me always to look to You for my answers and not to other things. Teach me to use food in the way You designed it to be used in my life. I praise You for your forgiveness and Your help. Amen.

Today's Food Choices

(List all the foods you've eaten today)

_____

_____

_____

_____

Thoughts on Paper (Daily Journal Entry)

About to Pop

Tickler
My doctor told me to stop having intimate dinners for four.
Unless there are three other people.
Orson Welles

Tidbit
Did You Know?

"Sixty-eight percent of all Americans are overweight, and the percent-age of adults who are obese has been rising for a decade. Approximately 2–3 percent of Americans suffer from extreme or 'morbid' obesity, for which surgical treatment is recommended."[7]

Trap

Large portions.

Restaurants today have taken to plopping extraordinarily large portions of food onto our plates, and we have followed suit at home. We need to train ourselves to eyeball our portions and not exceed what we really need.

Trick
Make a change—switch to diet sodas, coffee, or tea sweetened with artificial sweetener like Splenda or others.

Did you know that eating one tiny piece of dark chocolate a day could actually benefit your health? Eating chocolate releases endorphins and causes you to feel better. Just be sure to eat only one small piece, and choose your time carefully.

Testimony

One day the truth dawned on me. Realizing that my mind leaks like a sieve, I decided I needed a reminder that consistent over-eating is a sin. The sin's name is Gluttony, and it's not God urging me to indulge in the mindless, greedy pleasure of overeating. I put a Post-it note, reading, "Gluttony comes from Satan!" on my computer monitor to remind me of that fact.

Beth Ann Ziarnik

Treasure

Give us today our daily bread.
MATTHEW 6:11

Thought for the Day

The Old Testament laws dictated certain requirements for eating and preparing food, but there is little mention in the New Testament about particular foods. Nevertheless, the New Testament indicates God's feelings on the matter of food consumption. He created food for our sustenance and for our enjoyment. The one sin mentioned in regard to food is gluttony, or overeating. Gluttons continue to eat even after they are full. Gluttony is the point at which food problems become spiritual problems. Eating a piece of cake or consuming a salty snack isn't necessarily sinful, but continuing to eat after you are full is clearly sinful. In God's eyes, being overweight isn't the root of the problem. He knows that all of our bodies are different and thus we carry our weight differently. Gluttony, however, is forbidden. Eating after you're already full is a real problem, especially for emotional eaters.

Keep canned tuna (the pop-top kind) in your car
to give to homeless people. Canned fruits and bottled water
are also nice to have on hand for such occasions.

Trusting God

Lord, I have to admit that I overeat sometimes. I keep going even after
I'm full. I ask You to forgive me for this, Father, and help me to stop
when I should. I also ask You to fill the empty places in my heart so
that I don't reach out for food with false hope. Help me make better
choices. Amen.

Today's Food Choices

(List all the foods you've eaten today)

_____

_____

_____

_____

Thoughts on Paper (Daily Journal Entry)

_____

_____

_____

_____

_____

_____

C'mon, Now (You Know It's Time)

Tickler
You know it's time to diet when you push away from the table and the table moves.
Quoted in "The Cockle Bur"

Tidbit
Did You Know?

Nearly every weight-loss candidate has used these words: "*Tomorrow* I'm going to start eating right." But, as the Broadway character Annie reminds us, tomorrow is always a day away.

Trap

Eating too fast.

One of the primary reasons we eat too much is simply because we eat too rapidly. We need to slow down and savor every bite. It takes about twenty minutes to get that "full" feeling, so take your time!

Trick
Make a list of realistic changes you would like to see in your life. Place the list on your refrigerator door or your bedside table so you don't forget where you've put it. Review the list every day.

Oatmeal—the wonder food. Oatmeal is one of the best morning foods we can eat. It's loaded with fiber, low in calories and fat, and gets our metabolism going in the morning. Start your day with some oatmeal.

Testimony

At the age of twenty-two I was a size 12/14. I rationalized what I didn't want to take the time to fix. I woke up one morning disgusted with my body and decided to change. My eating habits completely changed. I drank a lot of water and ate healthy foods. The weight virtually fell off. Within four months, I had lost twenty-five pounds. I continued to work out. I have now lost a total of thirty-five pounds and wear a size 3/5. Not only did I like the way I looked better, I also felt so much better. It's amazing that Jesus cares about what we care about. He is so desperate to see our desires come true. I delighted myself in Him as I worked out and ate healthy, and He blessed me. He deserves the glory.

Kylie Smith

Treasure

*Therefore, since we are surrounded by
such a great cloud of witnesses,
let us throw off everything that
hinders and the sin that so easily entangles,
and let us run with perseverance the race marked out for us.*
HEBREWS 12:1

Thought for the Day

It is possible to honor the Lord with the vessel He's given you, even if you've never tried. It's not too late. Even if you've failed in this area before, take heart! God will give you a fresh start. He wants His very best for you, and that includes great health and a body that's fit and comfortable. The Lord will bless your efforts and you will gain strength, both inside and out, as a result. The time for change has come. C'mon! You can do it!

Do you have relatives you haven't spoken to in a while?
Call them today.

Trusting God

Lord, I'm ready to make a fresh start today. I place the past in the past where it belongs. I admit that I'm unable to do this on my own. I need Your help. Please remind me daily of Your love for me just as I am, but also remind me of Your desire to see things change in my life. Help me, Lord. Amen.

Today's Food Choices

(List all the foods you've eaten today)

_____

_____

_____

_____

Thoughts on Paper (Daily Journal Entry)

_____

_____

_____

_____

_____

_____

D-E-C-I-D-E:
Six Letters That Can
Change Your Life

Tickler
Diet is "Die" with a T.
Unknown

Tidbit
Did You Know?

Americans eat a lot of high-fat foods, desiring to put taste and convenience ahead of nutrition.[8]

Trap

"Sugar-free" labels.

Shopping for low-cal or low-carb foods can get confusing, especially at first glance. You read a "sugar-free" label and assume the item is "free" of calories, as well. Wrong. Sugar-free cookies and desserts often have as many calories as "sugar-full" items do. Diabetics are happy to have the alternative, but the rest of us might just as well take a nibble of the real thing.

Trick
Wear snug clothes when you eat. This may sound funny, but it works. We're more aware of how much we eat when we can feel our clothes, especially around the waistline. Wearing loose-fitting clothes causes us to forget how much we're eating, but wearing a snug skirt or slacks will remind us throughout the meal that we need to take it easy.

Tangelos. Did you know they are half tangerine, half grape-fruit? Tangelos are loaded with vitamins and make a healthy, tasty snack.

Testimony

I decided I needed to come to the place where I chose God over food. So I literally gave my body to Him. From that point on, I decided I would eat nothing He didn't indicate He wanted me to eat. I considered myself "dead." Being "dead," I didn't need to eat any more. Being "dead," I didn't have to worry about whether or not I was fat. If God wanted me fat, so be it. If He wanted me to lose, that was up to Him. So I prayed with a friend to commit to this. At mealtime, I stood in front of the refrigerator and asked God if He wanted me to eat any-thing. If the answer in my heart was no, I ran from the kitchen as if it were on fire.

Beth Ann Ziarnik

Treasure

You were bought at a price.
Therefore honor God with your body.
1 CORINTHIANS 6:20

Thought for the Day

One decision can change your life. We discovered this when we came to the decision to trust the Lord and place our lives in His hand. One tiny decision can steer us to the right or to the left. That's why it's so important to make a decision—one you can stick with—regard-ing your eating habits. Years of nondecision can often lead to apathy or a feeling of hopelessness. But it's not too late. You can still decide. Decide to do something about your health today. Don't wait. Once you've made that decision, your body will follow suit. You might be surprised how difficult it isn't, once your mind is made up.

Been putting off a visit to your doctor, optometrist, or other professional? Make that appointment today.

Trusting God

Lord, today is the day I'm making a decision to change the rest of my life. I consciously choose to follow You and Your plan for my life. This includes my habits and my patterns of eating. Have Your will in me, Father. Keep me strong in You. Amen.

Today's Food Choices

(List all the foods you've eaten today)

_____

_____

_____

_____

Thoughts on Paper (Daily Journal Entry)

_____

_____

_____

_____

_____

_____

_____

Speak to the Mountain

Tickler

It isn't the mountain ahead that wears you out,
it's the grain of sand in your shoe.
Robert Service

Tidbit
Did You Know?

A survey by Roper Starch Worldwide shows that breakfasts, lunches, and dinners at the dining table are quickly becoming a thing of the past. The survey declared that most Americans eat all day long! Americans seemingly eat in their cars, at the ballpark, and in front of their computers.[9]

Trap

Eating out.

When you eat out, you are far more likely to consume extra calories and carbohydrates. Even foods from the "healthy menu" often are cooked in butter or oil. Restaurants are notorious for serving double-sized portions, so if you must eat out, tell yourself that you will only eat half of what's on your plate.

Trick

Stop looking at food as your enemy. All foods were given to us to enjoy. You can't look at a particular food as "good" or "bad." When you feel like eating a food you really enjoy, go ahead. Just eat it slowly and try to stop at the halfway point. That way, you really can have your cake and eat it, too!

Treat

Treat your sweet tooth to a half-cup of sherbet. It's low in fat and calories and satisfies the craving for something sweet and delicious.

Testimony

The funniest thing that happened to me was one time when my scale got stuck. I was distressed that I was trying so hard and thought I was thinner judging from my clothes, yet the scale stayed the same. I'd been on a medicine for my glaucoma that made me gain weight, so I was doubly distressed. I found myself angry with God for letting this happen to me. My faith was pretty shaky at the time, due to other things. Then I went to the doctor because I'd slipped and fallen, and I discovered that I'd actually lost eleven pounds. My scale at home was stuck. I hope God just laughed at me. I felt chagrined for being upset with Him.

Laurie Alice Eakes

Treasure

*He replied, "Because you have so little faith.
I tell you the truth, if you have faith as small as a mustard seed,
you can say to this mountain, 'Move from here to there'
and it will move. Nothing will be impossible for you."*
MATTHEW 17:20

Thought for the Day

How many times do we look at the mountains in our way and give up before the journey begins? "I can't lose weight, because my family won't support me." "I can't conquer this demon, because I have to eat out every day." "I'll never be able to do this, because I've been overweight all my life." On and on the list goes.

Don't be tricked into believing your weight is the enemy or that you can't overcome daily obstacles. They are nothing in comparison to our powerful God. Ask the Lord for an increase of faith regarding your eating habits. With His help, those mountains have no choice but to move out of the way!

· · · · · · · · · (Turning Your Focus) · · · · · · · · · · · ·

Have a special hobby?
Consider joining a group of like-minded folks in your area.

Trusting God

Father, I have to admit that I've been looking at the mountains in my life—the foods I love, the meals out, my extra pounds—and seeing them as impossible to overcome. Today, I speak to those mountains. Help me to see that for You even a mountain is no problem. Amen.

Today's Food Choices

(List all the foods you've eaten today)

_____

_____

_____

_____

Thoughts on Paper (Daily Journal Entry)

Day 10

Forgetting the Fads

Tickler
A diet is the penalty we pay for exceeding the feed limit.
Author Unknown

Tidbit
Did You Know?

Extreme dieting poses dangers. Not only that, but statistics also show that 80 to 90 percent of dieters regain the weight they lost.[10]

> ### Trap
>
> Trying to lose weight quickly.
>
> It will surely come back just as quickly. I can't emphasize how important this is. You will stand a better chance of keeping the weight off if you lose it slowly. Don't be discouraged at a weight loss of only a pound or two a month. By the end of the year, you'll be twelve to twenty-four pounds lighter, and you will probably stay that way!

Trick
Create a new motto for yourself: "Never do today what you're not willing to do for the rest of your life." Then, whenever you're tempted to "fad diet," you'll always be reminded that you couldn't possibly keep it up for the rest of your life. Take one day at a time.

Testimony

I did extreme things to get thin. Starving myself, exercising excessively, and even abusing laxatives. You name it, I tried it. I wanted desperately to get control of the monster that raged within me. I have found out only recently that it is only God who can squelch this monster, and only if I daily submit myself to His care and will.

Mary Hanlon

Treasure

In his heart a man plans his course,
but the LORD determines his steps.
PROVERBS 16:9

Thought for the Day

Never do today what you're unwilling to do for the rest of your life. For me, that meant I couldn't do any high-speed dieting. I couldn't commit to eating grapefruit every day for the rest of my life. I couldn't commit to eating large quantities of meat every day for the rest of my life. I couldn't commit to drinking liquid meals every day for the rest of my life. You get the point. My plan would have to be something sensible that I could keep up with. Forever. Like it or not, my "diet" would truly last the rest of my life. I could only live with that if I chose the correct plan for me.

Work on your photo album
or make an album for a family member.

Trusting God

Lord, I have to admit I often fall into the trap of thinking I have to "fad" diet in order to lose weight quickly. I've purchased products that didn't do any good. I've eaten so-called healthy foods in excess, but I haven't really learned to live in balance. Help me in this area, Lord. I want to lose weight, but I want to do it Your way. Amen.

Today's Food Choices

(List all the foods you've eaten today)

_____

_____

_____

_____

Thoughts on Paper (Daily Journal Entry)

_____

_____

_____

_____

_____

_____

_____

The Cost of Eating Right

Tickler
Things sweet to taste prove.in digestion sour.
William Shakespeare

Tidbit
Did You Know?

Forty billion dollars are spent by Americans each year on dieting and diet-related products.[12]

(Trap)

"Diet" pills.

All you have to do is turn on the television to hear the promotional ads for the latest diet pills. They promise fast, permanent weight loss. They make guarantees—and, out of desperation, we believe them. Don't be fooled. Weight loss is not found in a pill. Marketers of dieting pills are only interested in one thing—making money from your vulnerability. And they don't mind doing it at great risk to your health. Don't buy into their trap. If you do, you will find your money swiftly floating down the drain and your health compromised.

Trick

Purchase a large bag of mixed fruit instead of chips or cookies. You'll spend about the same amount of money but come home with a much better deal.

-------------------------------(Treat)-------------------------------

Did you know that those inexpensive, low-calorie, low-fat containers of yogurt can be frozen? For a yummy snack, place your favorite flavor in the freezer for one hour. Be sure to give it a good stir before eating.

Testimony

I have learned that creating a weekly meal plan helps not only my eating habits but also my pocketbook. When I construct a realistic menu at the beginning of the week, I only purchase foods from the list. This helps me when I shop. It also helps me when I feel like snacking. It's hard to eat something that's not there!

Janice Thompson

Treasure

And do not set your heart on what
you will eat or drink;
do not worry about it.
For the pagan world runs after all such things,
and your Father knows that you need them.
But seek his kingdom,
and these things will be given to you as well.
LUKE 12:29–31

Thought for the Day

When you set out on the road to lose weight and get in shape, you have to be prepared to spend a little money. Eating right isn't cheap. Of course, neither are boxes of chocolates, Rocky Road ice cream, and potato chips. Boneless chicken breasts and fresh fruit now take the place of those things, and though they cost a little more, they're worth it. Eating healthy is more expensive, but in the long run, you will discover it is far cheaper and less painful than obesity, heart problems, high cholesterol, and other weight-related health problems.

Turning Your Focus

If you have a friend who's struggling with an illness, cook him or her a meal.

Trusting God

Lord, I know You see my need for financial provision and good health. Help me to overcome this nagging doubt that getting into shape is going to be too costly. Help me plan carefully, implement strategically, and live faithfully. Amen.

Today's Food Choices

(List all the foods you've eaten today)

_____

_____

_____

_____

Thoughts on Paper (Daily Journal Entry)

Doctor, Doctor

Tickler
The cardiologist's diet: If it tastes good, spit it out.
Author Unknown

Tidbit
Did You Know?

Obesity-related diseases annually cost Americans an estimated $120 billion. Obesity and other weight-related problems have overtaken smoking and are now the single most preventable cause of illness and death in the U.S.[13]

Trap

Caffeine.

People everywhere are addicted. They can't go a day without caffeine for fear of migraines. But why? With so many caffeine-free products available, why would people still turn to this stimulant? Like many other substances, it is addictive and difficult to overcome. Giving it up—at least in large quantities—is recommended. Excessive caffeine intake can interrupt your ability to focus, speed up your heart rate, and actually stir up false hunger pangs.

Trick

Losing even 10 percent of your current weight can substantially improve your health. Sleep apnea, high cholesterol, and high blood pressure might all be affected by a minimal weight loss. Set small goals and watch your health improve.

Treat

Watermelon is a magic fruit—a natural diuretic that is loaded with vitamins. It is also high in fiber, low in calories, and nearly devoid of fat. It is sweet, filling, and delicious. When you purchase a watermelon, cut it into small pieces and place in handy containers. That way, when your sweet tooth begs for something delicious, you'll be ready.

Testimony

I went to the doctor for a check-up and he told me I needed to "drop a few pounds." This was an understatement, because I needed to drop about seventy-five pounds. I sighed and replied, "Yeah, I know." His response: "You don't seem surprised." What does he think, that I don't look in the mirror every morning?

Mary Walton

Treasure

Dear friend, I pray that you may enjoy good health
and that all may go well with you,
even as your soul is getting along well.
3 JOHN 1:2

Thought for the Day

Speak to your doctor. With his or her help, select a diet that is sensible and workable for you. For many, a low-calorie, low-fat, high-fiber diet is the key. Lean meats, such as chicken and fish, combined with fruits, vegetables, and grains, will increase your energy level and give you the vitamins and minerals you need to keep going. Let your doctor monitor your progress. Be prepared for some basic tests on your thyroid and liver as you begin.

· · · · · · · · · · · · · · (Turning Your Focus) · · · · · · · · · · · · · ·

Send a funny online card to someone who's feeling blue.

Trusting God

Lord, I pray that You will help me overcome the fear of facing my doctor with my weight problem. Help me overcome the fear of stepping on the scale. Give me the courage to ask my doctor for help and advice. I need courage and wisdom, Lord. Amen.

Today's Food Choices
(List all the foods you've eaten today)

_____

_____

_____

_____

Thoughts on Paper (Daily Journal Entry)

_____

_____

_____

_____

_____

Mission, Possible!

Tickler

Losing weight is a triumph of mind over platter.
Anonymous

Tidbit

Did You Know?

" 'No pain, no gain' is not always true. If exercise is too strenuous, you may dread doing it and therefore put it off until you finally give it up entirely."[14]

Trap

Battered and fried.

You see it everywhere. Chicken-fried steak. Chicken-fried chicken. Battered and fried okra, tomatoes, etc. Perfectly good food smothered in flour and milk and deep-fried in oil. Though these foods might taste great, they are high in fat, loaded with calories and carbs, and tough on the arteries. Try cooking your meats and vegetables without all the added junk—by grilling, steaming, or broiling. Your body will thank you.

Trick

Eat breakfast. Did you realize that skipping breakfast causes your body to remain in "storing fat" mode? When you take that first bite in the morning, the storage stops and your metabolism gets a jolt.

Testimony

After one-and-a-half weeks of low-carb dieting, I had to have some pizza. There's only so much steak and sausage and eggs and bacon that you can eat before pizza calls out your name. It is a lot easier to get by now, because I have discovered sugar-free desserts. But for some reason, they make me want the real thing. I also sneak one bite of spaghetti from my wife when she lets me. But it seems the world is becoming more and more weight-loss friendly, so I am going to stick with it for a while and see how well I can do.

Zachary Morrow

Treasure

Now the Lord is the Spirit,
and where the Spirit of the Lord is, there is freedom.
2 CORINTHIANS 3:17

Thought for the Day

Choose a logical plan. Part of the reason we fail at losing weight and getting into shape is simply because we don't have a strategy. We need guidance from the Lord, and we need to reason with ourselves. What is realistic? Can we keep up with whatever plan we have chosen? Can we afford it? How will others in the family react? Will we be able to eat out on occasion? If we take the time to think these things through in advance, we'll stand a far greater chance of seeing things through till the end.

Trusting God

Lord, today I ask for guidance from You. I need to know Your opinion. Give me vision and clarity and help me implement the plan that You have for me. Father, I don't want my eating habits to be chaotic. I need structure and order in this area. Help me move forward with Your plan in mind. Amen.

Today's Food Choices

(List all the foods you've eaten today)

_____

_____

_____

_____

Thoughts on Paper (Daily Journal Entry)

_____

_____

_____

_____

_____

_____

_____

Flying Solo

Tickler

It is a hard matter, my fellow citizens,
to argue with the belly, since it has no ears.
Plutarch

Tidbit

Did You Know?

If you feel depressed about your body, or if you start bingeing or fasting, then getting professional help is a good idea. Counselors and psychologists trained in the areas of body image can guide you in changing negative beliefs and behaviors. If you are a chronic crash-dieter, you might need assistance from a dietician or a psychologist who can introduce healthier ways of eating and help you improve how you relate to and care for your body.[15]

Trap

Pride.

One of the weaknesses we face is our own pride. We don't tell anyone that we're trying to cut back, in case we fail. If we fail alone, no one has to know. But acquiring and keeping a good support system is critical when setting out on the road to a healthy lifestyle. We need one another too much to fly solo.

Trick

Make one change at a time. For example, if you usually drink three sodas a day, try cutting back to two.

····················(Treat)····················

Toast a piece of wheat bread and put a small amount of apple butter or sugar-free jelly on it. This yummy treat is almost as good as a cinnamon roll.

Testimony

I was finally going to do it right. I'd started a hundred diets before, but this time I was going to get serious. They always tell you to consult your physician before beginning any weight-loss program, so I made an appointment with a clinic and was assigned to a doctor I'd never met. When she came into the room, I saw that she weighed 300 pounds. When I asked her about a healthy, effective, sensible weight-loss plan, she said, "Eat less and exercise more." I was on my own.

Mary Connealy

Treasure

When Moses' hands grew tired,
they took a stone and put it under him and he sat on it.
Aaron and Hur held his hands up—
one on one side, one on the other—
so that his hands remained steady till sunset.
EXODUS 17:12

Thought for the Day

Remember the story of the Israelites battling the Amalekites? As the people faced their enemy, the Lord instructed Moses to lift his arms while the battle was being fought. After a while, he grew weary and his arms fell to his side. When that happened, the Israelites began to lose the battle. Other men of God came rushing to Moses' side and held his arms up for him. Together, they managed to garner the strength to see the battle won. Regardless of what plan we choose or what foods we prefer, we simply can't do this weight-loss thing alone. We need the Lord. We also need one another. With so many people trying to get in shape, finding a weight-loss buddy won't be difficult. Look around your community for a regular meeting, or turn to the Internet for a support group. Also, while you're seeking the assistance of others, don't be ashamed or embarrassed to contact a nutritionist. A skilled dietician will be able to help you with meal planning, calorie counting, and a host of other things.

Turning Your Focus

Ask your pastor if there's anything you can do
to help at the church today.

Trusting God

Lord, I pray that you will send just the right people to lift my arms during this journey to get in shape. I need encouragers, Lord. Also, help me to be an encouragement to others. May we, together, look to You for the answers we need. Amen.

Today's Food Choices
(List all the foods you've eaten today)

_____

_____

_____

_____

Thoughts on Paper (Daily Journal Entry)

The Ride Begins

Tickler

*Probably nothing in the world arouses more false hopes
than the first four hours of a diet.*
Dan Bennett

Tidbit

Did You Know?

When you've gotten yourself all mixed up by using external rules to
guide your eating (i.e., dieting), it takes a little while to get back on
track.[16]

> ·············(**Trap**)·················
>
> Seconds.
>
> In our fast-paced world, we often eat so quickly that we don't
> fill up right away. Still feeling hungry, we sometimes reach for
> seconds. But instead of filling up our plates again, we should
> slow down and take time for the hunger pangs to dissipate. If
> we do, we'll find that firsts are quite enough.

Trick

I've found that eating from a smaller plate helps a lot.
Lena Nelson Dooley

Testimony

I started my first diet at age fifteen when my father promised he'd buy me a car if I dropped twenty-five pounds. I lost that twenty-five pounds and auditioned for a school play. I was given one of the leads in the production and had the time of my life. I'll never forget the feeling of exhilaration that came with being a "new person." Losing those pounds gave me the courage to try something I had never tried before and motivated me to do more than ever before.

Janice Thompson

Treasure

The Lord does not let the righteous go hungry
but he thwarts the craving of the wicked.
PROVERBS 10:3

Thought for the Day

There is nothing more exciting than the first few days of healthy eating. The first pounds often fly off, which can be an exhilarating boost to the ego. Remember, the thrill of the journey will not always be this high. Things will not always go as well and your desire will ebb and flow. You will encounter days when you feel like giving up. However, you must never forget the feeling you had the first time you stepped on the scale and saw a lower number, or slipped on a pair of pants and didn't have to strain to get them zipped. That first exciting bit of weight loss can be a tremendous motivator for the rest of the journey.

Turning Your Focus

Tired of the same old thing?
Consider rearranging the furniture
in one of the rooms of your home.

Trusting God

Lord, I thank You for the enthusiasm to begin this journey. I couldn't do it without You. I pray that You will remind me, when things are a little tougher, that You have been with me every step of the way. Amen.

Today's Food Choices

(List all the foods you've eaten today)

_____

_____

_____

_____

Thoughts on Paper (Daily Journal Entry)

_____

_____

_____

_____

_____

_____

_____

Charting the Course

Tickler

In the Middle Ages, they had guillotines,
stretch racks, whips, and chains.
Nowadays, we have a much more effective torture device
called the bathroom scale.
Stephen Phillips

Tidbit
Did You Know?

Most weight-loss diets provide 1,000 to 1,500 calories per day. However, the right number of calories for you depends on your weight and activity level.[17]

··(Trap)························

Eating too little.

Let's face it; sometimes we eat too little in order to overcompensate for the times we've eaten too much. We figure the fast-after-feasting method is best. The only problem with this approach is that we need a more stable plan. Starving ourselves today only makes us hungrier tomorrow. Of course, there are occasionally times when the Lord calls us to a biblical fast. Just make sure you're hearing from Him before you decide to go without eating.

Trick

Keep a weight-loss journal. You'll be surprised at how your willpower grows when you have to write down everything you've eaten.

··············· (Treat) ···············

Green beans are quite low in calories (just 43.75 calories in a whole cup) and are loaded with enough nutrients to not only power up the Jolly Green Giant but also put a big smile on his face. Green beans are an excellent source of fiber and vitamins K and A, and a very good source of vitamin C, riboflavin, potassium, iron, manganese, folic acid, magnesium, and thiamin.[18]

Testimony

I will testify to the wisdom of losing weight slowly—you keep it off. When you're small, you always think that you're bigger than you are. When I was twenty-six, I gained thirty pounds in three months. I started journaling, watching my habits. What was I eating? When? In my case a good friend was "feeding" me gourmet foods (her treat to me). I started an exercise regime. I exercised and didn't lose a pound. But I had read an article about muscle mass. After that year, I lost forty pounds in six months. I figured out how to eat and what level of exercise was good for me.

Denise McEwen

Treasure

For it is we who are the circumcision,
we who worship by the Spirit of God,
who glory in Christ Jesus,
and who put no confidence in the flesh—
though I myself have reasons for such confidence.
PHILIPPIANS 3:3–4

71

Thought for the Day

Keep a journal of your food intake and your daily activities. This simple step will motivate you and let you look back over the months to see how far you've come. I created a database on my computer with several columns. The last column—Notes—is filled with priceless jottings that still make me smile. In that column I wrote personal things that happened in my day, both good and bad, and listed the things God was doing in my life. I still laugh and cry when I go back to read those entries.

.... (Turning Your Focus) ....

Set a date to visit a local museum with a loved one.

Trusting God

Lord, I thank You that You know every step of my journey, even before I take it. Help me to chart Your course, not my course, and give me the courage to walk it out, day by day. Amen.

Today's Food Choices

(List all the foods you've eaten today)

_____

_____

_____

_____

Thoughts on Paper (Daily Journal Entry)

_____

_____

_____

_____

_____

_____

_____

_____

_____

_____

_____

_____

_____

_____

_____

_____

_____

_____

_____

Small Goals

Tickler
Habit is a habit and not to be flung out of the window by any man but coaxed downstairs a step at a time.
Mark Twain

Tidbit
Did You Know?

According to the National Institutes of Health, a reasonable weight-loss goal is one or two pounds per week for a period of six months, with the subsequent strategy based on the amount of weight lost.[19]

Trap

Sugary breakfasts.

Sweet breakfast cereals, cinnamon rolls, toaster treats, and other early morning goodies might sound tempting, but the initial sugar high they supply will usually cause you to "crater" a short time later. For a high-energy day, stay away from sugar, particularly early in the morning.

Trick
Use the bathroom scale only once a week. Your weight fluctuates too much to stress yourself out over the ups and downs of a daily weigh-in. Besides, how you look and feel may be a more reliable indicator than your weight.

Testimony

I had a hard time making the decision and commitment to change my eating habits, even though I knew I seriously needed to. Then one day my doctor called to tell me I had a major yeast imbalance and must cut out all sugar and severely limit starchy foods if I wanted to get my health back in balance. It's funny sometimes how the Lord works. I guess this was a good kick in the pants to get going and make the changes I needed to make.

Carrie Turansky

Treasure

And lead us not into temptation, but deliver us from the evil one.
MATTHEW 6:13

Thought for the Day

Sometimes, we bite off a little more than we can chew (pardon the pun), especially when it comes to controlling our weight. We decide to take off a few pounds, and we're convinced we can do it quickly and effectively, so we rapidly jump into the latest plan of action. Unfortunately, we often try to do too much too quickly. We want to lose a lot of weight—fast. We want to fit into a new swimsuit in a couple of weeks. We want to impress an old friend we haven't seen in years. It takes a while to figure out that getting into shape takes time. If we set small, attainable goals, we will be more likely to achieve them. Setting large, unrealistic goals is a surefire setup for failure.

(Turning Your Focus)

Go through your books and give away ones you've
already read to a homeless shelter, retirement home,
or other organization where they'll be put to good use.

Trusting God

Father, I need wisdom to know what sort of goals I should set for myself when it comes to realistic weight loss. Help me to know the difference between realistic and unrealistic. Give me the strength I need
to admit that I can't do this in a hurry. I need Your help, Lord. Amen.

Today's Food Choices
(List all the foods you've eaten today)

_____

_____

_____

_____

Thoughts on Paper (Daily Journal Entry)

_____

_____

_____

_____

_____

_____

Lite Support

Tickler
*As for food, half of my friends have
dug their graves with their teeth.*
Chauncey M. Depew

Tidbit
Did You Know?

According to a report in the Journal of the American Medical Association, weight-loss efforts can be helped through the Internet. Researchers studying a group of ninety-one overweight hospital employees for
six months found that group therapy, provided by means of an e-mail
newsletter, discussion forum, and individualized therapist feedback
through the Internet, achieved a 5 percent reduction of weight.[21]

Trap

Cooking for the family.

It is possible to garner the support you need, even from your
family. When cooking meals for the home crew, just be sure
to prepare menus in advance and stick to them. Don't veer
from your original plan, even when your loved ones are beg-
ging for sugary substitutes.

Trick

Here's a little trick that's sure to keep you on your toes, as well as make you accountable. Share the experience of eating right with a friend who is attempting to do the same thing. Check in with each other at least once a day, and send a list of what you've eaten to each other, if this will motivate you further.

Treat

Treat yourself to membership in a local weight-loss group. Join a support group near your home and hang out with like-minded folks who desire to eat right and improve their health. This little treat is sure to lift your spirits and keep you motivated to do the right thing.

Testimony

I've noticed how our church does a lot around food. Whether it's always giving the little ones snacks in the nursery or children's church, the weekly donut time before adult Sunday school, or the finger foods at all the youth group gatherings, I don't know if it's such a good pattern to follow. Families sign up to bring treats, and it doesn't always have to be pastries—some people have brought rolls or fruit or juice—but it's amazing how the cream-filled stuff always seems to show up. I worry sometimes that we are abusing our temples in the name of fellowship. We say we should honor God, and we preach against the sins of back-biting, gossip, anger, disobedience, and so on, but what about gluttony? What are we doing to ourselves?

Lynette Sowell

Treasure

Therefore encourage each other with these words.
1 Thessalonians 4:18

Thought for the Day

Support is critical to getting into shape. We need the help of our friends, family, and fellow healthy eaters. We need the encouragement of others who are trying to do what we're doing—get in shape and improve our health. Some "life support" ideas include the following: Join a local support group and an online group (if you're Internet savvy). The online group will give you something the local group cannot—daily, minute-by-minute encouragement and advice. There are some amazing places online to help you keep track of your BMI (Body Mass Index) and daily calorie/carbohydrate intake. (www.fitday. com is one of my favorites!)

······· (Turning Your Focus) ···········
Purchase a small, unexpected gift for a loved one.
Wrap it in beautiful wrapping paper with ribbons and bows.

Trusting God

Father, thank You for bringing people into my life who can support my decision to be healthy. I pray that You would cause people to understand Your plan for my life so that they can support my decision to get in shape. Thank You, Lord, for sending people to minister to me during this crucial time. Amen.

Today's Food Choices

(List all the foods you've eaten today)

_____

_____

_____

_____

Thoughts on Paper (Daily Journal Entry)

_____

_____

_____

_____

_____

_____

_____

_____

_____

_____

_____

_____

_____

_____

_____

_____

_____

_____

_____

Craving, Temptation, Addiction

Tickler

If you have formed the habit of checking on
every new diet that comes along,
you will find that, mercifully, they all blur together,
leaving you with only one definite piece of information:
french-fried potatoes are out.
Jean Kerr

Tidbit
Did You Know?

In 1999, U.S. soft drink sales totaled $58 billion.[22]

Trap

Fast food.

In this modern, rush-about world, it is often easier to "pick up a bite to eat" on your way home from work (or the soccer game or PTA meeting) than to cook at home. Eating out isn't always the healthiest choice, but even fast food restaurants are getting into the swing of things by offering low-fat, higher fiber food choices. If you must drive through, be sure to order something a little healthier than burgers and fries.

Trick

This is an old trick, but a good one. Find a photo of yourself that will inspire you to lose weight. This might be a picture of yourself at a younger age and lower weight or it might be an image of yourself at a high weight. Either way, place it on the refrigerator door with a magnet and you'll be reminded to stick to your guns before you open the door.

······· (Treat) ···············

Treat yourself to a homemade smoothie. Combine frozen strawberries, half a banana, and some diet strawberry lemonade (or raspberry ice). Blend until smooth and creamy.

Testimony

After learning I had diabetes, I found that the best tip when grocery shopping is not to buy the tasty little tidbits I wanted. My mom lives with me, and her Alzheimer's makes her crave sweets. I still buy sweets, but I choose kinds I'm not crazy about. It's a constant battle. I also try to shop on the perimeter of the grocery store, where the fresh fruit is.

Eileen Key

Treasure

This is what the Lord says to you:
"Do not be afraid or discouraged because of this vast army.
For the battle is not yours, but God's."
2 CHRONICLES 20:15

Thought for the Day

Temptations abound. All you have to do is turn on the television, and you're inundated with commercials for tasty treats. Driving down the road, you face the challenge of delectable goodies at every turn. What's a person to do? How can you possibly continue to resist when "the good stuff" is staring you in the face every time you turn around?

First, you must acknowledge that food is not the enemy. One of the reasons we're so tempted to "cheat" is because of our ongoing "feast or fast" mentality. Instead of giving up every yummy thing, have a little bit of something you love every now and then. That way you won't be so tempted to swallow down large portions of high-fat goodies when you do take a tumble. Also, if you're especially tempted by sweets, try keeping ample portions of fruit in the house. Fruit is far better for you and it pacifies your sweet tooth.

· · · · · · · · · · · · (Turning Your Focus) · · · · · · · · · · · ·

Write a poem and give it to a friend or loved one.

Trusting God

Father, I know that with Your help I will never be tempted beyond that which I'm able to resist. Help me to resist giving in to an overabundance of poor food choices. Help me overcome my addictions, I pray. I give those things over to You, Lord. Amen.

Today's Food Choices

(List all the foods you've eaten today)

_____

_____

_____

_____

Thoughts on Paper (Daily Journal Entry)

Get a Move On!

Tickler
Never eat more than you can lift.
Miss Piggy

Tidbit
Did You Know?

According to Dr. Julie Gerberding, director of the Centers for Disease Control, "It is important for adults to get a minimum of thirty minutes of moderate physical activity most days of the week to help prevent chronic diseases and promote health."[23]

Trap

Fruit juices.

Despite the health benefits associated with fruit juices, they are often loaded with sugar, calories, and carbohydrates. Drink them in moderation.

Trick
Go out of your way. Park your car a block or two away from your destination and walk.

Testimony

If I don't exercise, I don't lose weight at all and I tend to over-eat. I can still ride my bike, but walking is best for me. At age 67, I've lost bone mass in my hip and lower back, according to my latest bone scan. The doctor said that walking and more calcium are the solutions. Being a type-A personality, my goal is not to look like my grandmother, who had obvious osteoporosis.

Martha Rogers

Treasure

I have no greater joy than to hear that my children walk in truth.
3 JOHN 1:4 NKJV

Thought for the Day

Exercise, but start slowly. Rome wasn't built in a day. Likewise, a 275-pound body can't jog three miles a day or bounce up and down on an elliptical machine for hours on end. I had to start by walking. Slowly. Then, as the weight began to come off, I gradually picked up speed. I had to drop below the 200-pound mark before I felt comfortable joining a gym, which I recently did.

Turning Your Focus

Go above and beyond the call of duty for your boss today.

Trusting God

Lord, give me the strength to begin a reasonable exercise plan. Increase my motivation level, I pray. Give me the time and the resources necessary to accomplish the task You have set before me. Amen.

Today's Food Choices
(List all the foods you've eaten today)

_____

_____

_____

_____

Thoughts on Paper (Daily Journal Entry)

_____

_____

_____

_____

_____

_____

_____

_____

_____

_____

Well Done Is
Half Begun

Tickler
Life itself is the proper binge.
Julia Child

Tidbit
Did You Know?

"Even a small weight loss (10 percent of your current weight) lowers the risk of several diseases."[24]

(Trap)

Cutting back in front of others, bingeing when alone.

Trick
Don't let your weight or condition keep you from activities that you enjoy.[25]

Peaches and antioxidants? Dessert with this fleshy fruit is healthier than expected, researchers are finding. And even greater levels of cancer-fighting antioxidants and other phyto-chemicals will be typical for new peach varieties in coming years.[26]

Testimony

I'm at the point in this journey where I've decided I will not quit, regardless. If I fall, so what? God picks me up and I begin again. The huge difference between now and a few years ago is that now I care. It used to be I'd eat a whole cake (routinely, actually) and never think about it or feel bad afterward. I'd eat two or three helpings of dinner every night. I'd order a super-sized meal and never blink. All of this was just commonplace. Now I come under conviction because the Holy Spirit is chasing me down and reminding me that my level of accountability in this area is higher since God has revealed truth to me.

Janice Thompson

Treasure

Blessed is the man who perseveres under trial,
because when he has stood the test,
he will receive the crown of life that God has promised
to those who love him.
JAMES 1:12

Thought for the Day

Oh, the joy of losing those first few pounds. Oh, the satisfaction of knowing you're on your way. Oh, the frustration of secretly fighting the same old temptations. One of the hardest struggles at this point in the journey is the never-ending battle between right and wrong. The weight is coming off, and it's because you're doing things right. You're still struggling with old temptations and are tempted to do the wrong thing. Relax! Try to remember that every day is a journey of its own. You will make mistakes, but you can just as surely pick up the pieces and begin again tomorrow. Look how far you've come, after all!

Turning Your Focus

Perform a random act of kindness. . .in secret.

Trusting God

Lord, sometimes I feel as if I have such a long way to go to accomplish my goals. Don't ever let me forget all the work You've already done in me. Thank You for the things You've taught me already. Help me not to forget! Help me always to look ahead and not backward at the mistakes of the past. Amen.

Today's Food Choices

(List all the foods you've eaten today)

_____

_____

_____

_____

Thoughts on Paper (Daily Journal Entry)

ROUNDING THE TURN

"Nothing tastes
as good as
thin feels."
ANONYMOUS

As the horses barrel down the track, something amazing happens. Instead of losing steam, their stamina actually increases. At this point, they are not so much worried about leading the pack as surviving the journey. Therefore, they are content to let other horses whiz by to set the pace. Undaunted, they press ahead, knowing that sometimes it is the slower, steadier horse who eventually wins the race.

The same is true with weight loss. Tearing out of the gate, we press forward to win the prize. But somewhere along the way we discover that "pressing" is work, and we slow down a bit in order to catch our breath. We pace ourselves, realizing this is the safest way to actually make it to the finish line. And make it we must!

At this point, we are convinced that the journey won't be as tough as we feared. After all, the first twenty-one days are behind us now. We have formed a new habit. Healthy eating is now a lifestyle. What we do during this middle leg of the journey is as critical, however, as that initial decision to get in shape. We must use these next twenty-one days to draw closer to the Lord as He gives us the strength and the courage to continue running the race He has set before us.

Crossing the Jordan

Tickler
To make your dreams come true,
you have to stay awake.
Anonymous

Tidbit
Did You Know?

Over the years, the prevalence of overweight people has steadily increased among nearly every racial or ethnic group.[27]

___

Trap

The feeling that you are indestructible.

Though faith is a good thing, overwhelming confidence is not. Just at the time when you begin to think you're indestructible, the enemy could attack. Always be on guard!

___

Trick
Keep a small ice chest in the car with baggies full of mini carrots, grapes, apple slices, water, etc. Be prepared!
Laura Porter

Testimony

When I get home from work really hungry, I can get into eating all the wrong, easy-to-grab snacks while preparing supper. Here's one thing that has helped me avoid this trap: As soon as I get home, I make a dish of apple slices—one apple cut in half, center seed pocket removed with a melon scoop, and the halves sliced into several wedges each. It's a great healthy snack, only one point on the Weight Watchers Program, and popping a slice in my mouth here and there as I make supper calms my "food frenzy." Hey, and an apple a day keeps the doctor away. I can live with that!

Beth Ann Ziarnik

Treasure

*But your hearts must be fully committed to the LORD our God,
to live by his decrees and obey his commands, as at this time.*
1 KINGS 8:61

Thought for the Day

You've done it! You've crossed from one phase to the next. Congratulations! You have now formed a new habit. Remember when you were concerned that you couldn't change your eating habits? Remember when you simply didn't care how much food you consumed in a day? Thank goodness those days are behind you. You have rounded the curve in the road and are pressing forward to reach your goal. As you enter this second phase of getting into shape, remember that the Lord will sustain and strengthen you all the way. He is for you, not against you. Be encouraged and don't turn back, no matter what.

··········· (Turning Your Focus) ···············

Write the author of a favorite book,
telling him or her how much you enjoyed it.

Trusting God

Lord, I stand amazed when I think of how much my life has changed over the past three weeks. Thank You for giving me the courage to begin this new walk of faith. I need Your strength and Your courage to get through this second leg of the journey. I place my life—and this body—into Your hands. Amen.

Today's Food Choices
(List all the foods you've eaten today)

_____

_____

_____

_____

Thoughts on Paper (Daily Journal Entry)

_____

_____

_____

_____

_____

_____

_____

Photo Replay

Tickler
Instead of crying over spilt milk, go milk another cow.
Erna Asp

Tidbit
Did You Know?

The average bowling ball weighs eight to ten pounds. When you've lost a few pounds, you can tell yourself, "I've lost one bowling ball." Just think of how many bowling balls it would be if you lost forty or fifty pounds. (How could you possibly hold them all at once?)

Trap

Giving up when you've made a mistake.

How many times do we give up after stumbling a bit? We eat a chocolate chip cookie and decide the diet is over. We swallow a couple pieces of pizza and get so discouraged that we decide there's no way to climb back on the wagon. Our mistakes should propel us forward, make us more determined than ever. We can't give up!

Trick
Here's a trick that's sure to keep you out of trouble: Prepare your lunch the night before so you're ready to go in the morning. That way, you'll have a plan and won't cater to the temptation to "grab a bite" with the gang from the office.

Testimony

I have never been obese, but I have gained and lost fifty pounds at least four times in my life, and gained and lost lesser amounts the rest of the time. I was never at a steady weight, I was always on my way up or down. Like many women, I had a range of sizes in my closet. How much I weighed and which clothes I was wearing was the measure of my self-worth. This was before I knew the Lord.

Mary Hanlon

Treasure

Put on the new self,
created to be like God in true righteousness and holiness.
EPHESIANS 4:24

Thought for the Day

To keep from getting discouraged during this middle stage, look at how far you've come. Pull out an old photo of yourself and compare it with a current one. Go through your closet and give away some of those clothes that are too loose around the waistline. Remind yourself daily that you have made progress in spite of any defeats. Even if the weight isn't pouring off, your mind-set has changed and your will to win is stronger than ever. You have, after all, put on a new self. Your attitude has changed, but so has your desire to be more like the Lord. No surrender, no defeat!

Do you have a talent or ability you've neglected?
Consider polishing it up and using it once again.

Trusting God

Lord, I'm so grateful for the progress in my life over the past few weeks. Even if things aren't perfect. Even if I'm not exactly where I want to be, I thank You for bringing me this far. Help me to love the journey. Amen.

Today's Food Choices

(List all the foods you've eaten today)

_____

_____

_____

_____

Thoughts on Paper (Daily Journal Entry)

_____

_____

_____

_____

_____

_____

_____

Stop to Smell the Roses

Tickler

I am not a glutton—I am an explorer of food.
Erma Bombeck

Tidbit
Did You Know?

"Most overweight people have no more psychological problems than people of average weight."[28]

Trap

Excessive amounts of any one food.

Many fall into the trap of liquid diets or only eating one food. They consume seven grapefruits in one day and wonder why they can't seem to function. They eat nothing but salad for a week and wonder why they feel like eating everything in the house on the weekends. A good, healthy balance is the key when trying to lose weight. Any diet that forces you to consume too much of a particular food is only a temporary solution to an ongoing problem.

Trick
Spice is nice. If you like spicy foods but don't care for the fat or calories, try adding salsa to your low-cal or low-carb meal. It will really spice things up.

Testimony

I'd like to share with you some of the non-caloric-burning advantages of walking: (1) time to praise God for His beautiful works of creation; (2) time to intercede for those God brings to mind—whether a neighbor as you pass their house, someone who drives by, or even someone halfway around the world; (3) time to meditate on God's Word. (4) time to let your mind run wild with the imagination God has given you; (5) time to appreciate the sights, smells, and sounds of nature—crisp fallen leaves, the smell in the air after a rain, the chirping of the birds. Then, go back to number 1 and praise God all over again.

Rose Allen McCauley

Treasure

See how the lilies of the field grow.
They do not labor or spin.
MATTHEW 6:28

Thought for the Day

Relax! Don't take everything so seriously! Bask in the cool of the evening. Enjoy a sunset. Take a walk with someone you love. Don't get so caught up in the plan to lose weight that you forget to live. Jesus said that He came to give life—and that abundantly. In other words, life is meant to be lived to the fullest. Instead of fretting, try taking a few deep breaths and marveling in the beauty of the day.

Trusting God

Father, please don't let me ever forget to take time away from the busyness of my agenda. Keep my focus on You and not on my task. Give me the wisdom to know the difference between the two, and put continual words of praise on my lips. Amen!

Today's Food Choices

(List all the foods you've eaten today)

_____

_____

_____

_____

Thoughts on Paper (Daily Journal Entry)

_____

_____

_____

_____

_____

_____

_____

_____

It's Me, Oh Lord!

Tickler

Don't go out of your weigh to please anyone but yourself.
Author Unknown

Tidbit

Did You Know?

"Forty-six percent of nine- to eleven-year-olds are 'sometimes' or 'very often' on diets, and 82 percent of their families are 'sometimes' or 'very often' on diets."[29]

(Trap)

Focusing on your lack of willpower.

Remember, this journey to become healthy has nothing to do with your willpower. The battle is the Lord's.

Trick

To curb your appetite, drink a glass of water before you sit down to a meal.

Testimony

My best friend, Lori, and I were shopping for a purse for her to take on her honeymoon. We had both been really watching our calories and walking every day to be in fine form for her upcoming wedding. We were talking about how much weight we had lost and the lady at the purse counter overheard us. We told her we were looking for a purse and she asked what style. When Lori answered, the lady interjected, "If you want to look smaller, just carry a larger purse." Lori replied, "Can you tell me where the luggage department is?" You have to keep your sense of humor!

Janet Deslatte

Treasure

Each one should test his own actions.
Then he can take pride in himself,
without comparing himself to somebody else,
for each one should carry his own load.
GALATIANS 6:4–5

Thought for the Day

Do the very best job you can do. Don't compare your weight loss to that of others. This is not a race, nor is it a competition. You are an individual, with your own load to carry. Don't let others talk you into switching plans, unless you're already convinced in your heart you should be shifting gears. You and the Lord, together, make a great team. He will give you the direction, the encouragement, and the stamina. That's not to say you don't need others, but in the long run, they don't have to answer for your health. You do. Stay plugged in to

God and keep listening. He will reveal His truth about your situation. Be the individual you are.

. . . . (Turning Your Focus) . . . .

Locate an old friend you've lost track of and schedule a visit.

Trusting God

Lord, thank You for revealing Your truth to me. Help me not to compare myself to others or to worry about my plan versus their plans. Deliver me from the spirit of competition and help me see that You love me as the individual I am. Amen.

Today's Food Choices
(List all the foods you've eaten today)

_____

_____

_____

_____

Thoughts on Paper (Daily Journal Entry)

_____

_____

_____

_____

_____

Interior Design

Tickler

*If nature had intended our skeletons to be visible,
it would have put them on the outside of our bodies.*
Elmer Rice

Tidbit
Did You Know?

Food may seem an unlikely way to improve your mental health.
Yet, what you eat (or don't eat) can have a profound effect on your
emotional state. A number of other substances in foods may lessen
symptoms of depression by affecting brain chemicals.[30]

Trap

Convincing yourself you can never change.

Our enemy loves to hold us captive with the idea that we
can't change. He whispers in our ears, "Things will always
stay the way they are." But things can and do change. We can
and will change.

Trick
Make a big green salad for the main dish, with meat as the
"condiment."

> "The nutritional benefits of apple juice (as well as applesauce and many other apple products) are often underestimated because these foods are "quietly virtuous." It is what apple juice and other apple products don't contain (no fat, cholesterol or sodium) as well as what they do contain (in the way of newly discovered phytonutrients) that makes these well-liked foods an important part of a healthful dietary regimen."[31]

Testimony

Foods have "voices," but for some of us, no food has a stronger, more demanding or forceful voice than ice cream, especially triple chocolate. (This voice could mistakenly be called a craving by some.) As the ice cream's call for attention rang through my freezer door, mostly in the late evening, I could not coldly ignore it. A few summers ago, I soothed the ice cream voices for a gain of about fifteen pounds before I concluded this had to stop. Though I no longer keep ice cream in my home, even today when I am grocery shopping I must hurry by the ice cream section because I can still hear those voices calling me. The only answer is not to answer.

Rose McDowell

Treasure

Do not conform any longer to the pattern of this world,
but be transformed by the renewing of your mind.
Then you will be able to test and approve what God's will is—
his good, pleasing and perfect will.
ROMANS 12:2

Thought for the Day

Change is never easy, is it? How we are designed on the outside has been our primary focus for weeks, but the real change must come on the inside. God has designed us to crave Him, not food. This means that our focus must shift from food to Him. Sounds easy, but in the real world it's often more tempting to reach for something visible than to reach out to the Lord. He is calling us, wooing us, to do the right thing. Way down deep, in the interior of our souls, we can hear His call for change. Every day, we should draw closer to Him than the day before, until finally we hear His voice so clearly that we stop questioning.

Turning Your Focus

Tell a coworker what a great job he or she is doing today.

Trusting God

Father, I thank You that I am capable of change, with Your help. Change me on the inside first, Lord. Then help me do what You would have me do to change the outside. Remind me daily that what's on the inside matters more than what's on the outside. Amen.

Today's Food Choices

(List all the foods you've eaten today)

_____

_____

_____

_____

Thoughts on Paper (Daily Journal Entry)

_____

_____

_____

_____

_____

Step by Step

Tickler
Minutes at the table don't put on weight; it's the seconds.
Anonymous

Tidbit
Did You Know?

A single food is considered high in salt if it has 400 milligrams per serving or more of salt. One teaspoon of salt has 2,400 milligrams of sodium. Eating a lot of salt can lead to high blood pressure. High blood pressure can lead to a stroke or heart attack.[32]

Trap

Popcorn and a movie?

How often do we equate movie-going with nibbling? Unfortunately, the typical bag of movie popcorn has up to 800 calories and is loaded with salt. Talk about a crisis! If you have the munchies while in the theater, try nibbling on sunflower seeds or pieces of sugar-free candy instead.

Trick
Here's a small step toward success. Instead of salting your foods, trying adding other seasonings. Lemon juice, garlic, and fresh-ground pepper are just a few options.

Testimony

My hubby and I both have pe-
dometers that say "10K a Day." I
usually wear mine on the waist-
band of my pants, but I know
some people who wear them on
their shoes. A pedometer will
work on just about anything that
moves with each step you take.
I have found that on days that I
teach or watch my two preschool
granddaughters, I have no trouble
getting in the required steps or
more. But on days that are spent
mainly writing at my computer,
I have found that I need to walk
an extra two or three miles to get
my quota in. So, to aid in your
weight loss, take it one step at a
time—just make sure you take at
least ten thousand of them a day!

Rose Allen McCauley

Treasure

But as for you,
continue in what you have learned
and have become convinced of,
because you know those from whom you learned it.
2 TIMOTHY 3:14

Thought for the Day

Setting small goals is the key, especially when you have a lot of
weight to lose. Step by step, progress is made. Any big attempts to
lose quickly will surely fail, for weight lost quickly is always regained
quickly. When I started at 275 pounds, I knew that I had a long road
ahead of me. If I focus on my final goal (137.5 pounds—exactly half
my starting weight), I'd never make it. Instead, with my online group's
help, I set small goals (for example, by Valentine's Day, I'll weigh

this much; by Easter, I'll weigh this much; etc.). I still have a way to go, even as I write these words, but I'm learning to enjoy the journey.

····················(Turning Your Focus)··············

Know a couple with young children?
Why not give them a gift certificate for a night out?

Trusting God

Lord, I have to confess that part of the reason I don't reach my goals is because I struggle to set them in the first place. Help me to be a goal-setter, Lord. Give me the ability to see the goals and plans You have for me, then help me to accomplish those things in Your name. Amen.

Today's Food Choices
   (List all the foods you've eaten today)

_____

_____

_____

_____

Thoughts on Paper (Daily Journal Entry)

_____

_____

_____

_____

A Little Is a Lot

Tickler
*Another good reducing exercise consists in placing
both hands against the table edge and pushing back.*
Robert Quillen

Tidbit
Did You Know?

Portion sizes have increased two to five times over the original size for
the following popular foods:

Hershey's chocolate bar: 0.6 ounces in 1908 / 1.6–8.0 ounces in 2002

Burger King hamburger: 3.9 ounces in 1954 / 4.4–12.6 ounces in 2002

McDonald's soda: 7 fluid ounces in 1955 / 12–42 fluid ounces in
2002

Coca-Cola bottle: 6.5 fluid ounces in 1916 / 8–34 fluid ounces in
2002[34]

Trap

Long conversations over dinner.

Though these conversations can be enlightening and help
build relationships, at some point we should shift from the
dinner table to the living room so that our fingers don't keep
reaching for the goodies in front of us.

Trick

"Eat more, but eat less. Eat things that are bulky and full of fiber but lacking in calories."[35]

Testimony

When I was depressed about being overweight, I would sometimes call up my friends, those being the local food delivery people. And then sometimes, I would go out myself and gather up several other friends, those being ice cream and cookies, or a huge bag of burgers and fries from a drive-thru restaurant. I would immediately feel much better after a visit from these friends, but only for a few minutes. And then the depressed feelings came back, stronger than ever. I finally learned to replace my old friends with new friends, those who would be supportive, encouraging, and uplifting, and who could hug me back. From experience, I know that it's hard to hug a half-gallon of ice cream.

Gina Bishop

Treasure

They all ate and were satisfied,
and the disciples picked up twelve basketfuls
of broken pieces that were left over.
MATTHEW 14:20

Thought for the Day

Why do we eat so much? It's a puzzling question. We don't always eat to be satisfied. More often than not, we wolf down a ton of food in a hurry and don't get the sensation of being full until later. And the fast-food businesses know we're in a hurry. They cater to our speedy lives. They hand us huge portions, far larger than our parents or grand-parents would ever have considered eating. We not only eat those portions, but we also eat them quickly, not giving them time to fill us up before we're reaching for a dessert or a soda to chase them down. The next time you go to a fast-food restaurant, take a good long look at what you've been served. Then cut it in half and eat it as slowly as you can. A little certainly goes a long way.

Turning Your Focus

Give some thought to teaching or attending a Bible study.

Trusting God

Lord, forgive me for not paying attention to how much food I've eaten in the past. Help me to see that I don't need a massive amount of food to survive. I only need enough to make me healthy and strong. Give me wisdom in the moment, Lord. Amen.

Today's Food Choices

(List all the foods you've eaten today)

_____

_____

_____

_____

Thoughts on Paper (Daily Journal Entry)

_____

_____

_____

_____

_____

_____

_____

_____

_____

_____

_____

_____

_____

_____

_____

_____

_____

_____

_____

Shake It Till You Break It!

Tickler

*I have to exercise early in the morning
before my brain figures out what I'm doing.*
Anonymous

Tidbit
Did You Know?

One in five adults engage in high levels of activity, but one in four are largely inactive.[36]

Trap

Excesses.

One of the reasons we don't keep up with a stable exercise plan is because it isn't stable. Often, we dive into a program, trying to accomplish too much, too quickly. We want to work out an hour a day, every day. We tell ourselves we'll walk five miles on the first day and a little more each subsequent day. Setting realistic exercise goals is critical, because we won't keep it up if they're too extreme.

Trick
Walk your dog. Take Rover for a brisk walk on a beautiful day. He will love it and so will you. Enjoy the sunshine. Talk to a neighbor. Spend time in prayer.

Trying to lose weight? Reach for a cup of green tea instead of a diet beverage. Compared to caffeine or a placebo, consumption of green tea extract produced a significant 4 percent increase in 24-hour energy expenditure. If you consume 2,000 calories per day and don't gain or lose weight, an increase of 4 percent would translate roughly into an 80-calorie daily difference.[37]

Testimony

A few years ago, I decided I needed to lose a few pounds. I started right after Christmas, cutting back on my food intake. I didn't add any exercise. I was busy with work, kids, etc., and didn't think I had the time. For about four to six weeks, I didn't lose anything, although I was being careful about what I ate. I became frustrated, and started walking about an hour a day, and the weight started coming off. I realized that I have to combine healthy eating and exercise to get results.

Pam Hillman

Treasure

A cheerful look brings joy to the heart,
and good news gives health to the bones.
PROVERBS 15:30

Thought for the Day

Exercise is a critical part of any weight-loss regimen. It does what "cutting back" cannot—burns excess calories and develops muscle mass. It keeps us toned and energetic. But exercise does something else, as well. Exercise gives us the energy we need to get through our work-heavy days. Sounds crazy, doesn't it? In order to have more energy, we need to exercise? But it's true, especially for those who have sedentary jobs. Getting up on our feet energizes us and gives us strength for the tasks we must face.

Mow the neighbor's front yard after you finish your own.

Trusting God

Lord, when I don't feel like exercising, I pray that You will give me the "want to." Remind me that I'll feel better when I'm done. Take away the exhaustion so that I can begin with a renewed mind. Amen.

Today's Food Choices

(List all the foods you've eaten today)

_____

_____

_____

_____

Thoughts on Paper (Daily Journal Entry)

_____

_____

_____

_____

_____

_____

_____

_____

Sharp Mind

Tickler

Brain cells come and brain cells go,
but fat cells live forever.
Author Unknown

Tidbit

Did You Know?

Regular physical activity improves mood, helps relieve depression, and increases feelings of well-being. It can help control joint swelling and pain. "Physical activity of the type and amount recommended for health has not been shown to cause arthritis."[38]

Trap

Main courses.

Often our main courses are heavy in calories, carbs, and fat. We focus on the chicken-fried steak and forget about the salad and green beans. Next time, try a vegetable as the main course. If you must have a fried food, make sure it's a side dish and only take a tiny portion.

Trick

Try to limit the amount of highly processed foods you buy. They tend to contain more fat and salt.[39]

Testimony

I always feel good when I make the right food choices. It may be the choice to pass up a second helping. Or it may be the choice to choose a restaurant with a menu that gives me healthy choices. Or it may be the choice to have a small portion of birthday cake, and then make the choice to eat in moderation for the rest of the meal, and for the rest of the day.

Gina Bishop

Treasure

Choose my instruction instead of silver,
knowledge rather than choice gold,
for wisdom is more precious than rubies,
and nothing you desire can compare with her.
PROVERBS 8:10–11

Thought for the Day

How do we keep our minds sharp while cutting back on foods we love? It's really an opportunity to exercise mind over matter. When you're faced with options, choose the healthier one. When you're faced with temptation, take the time to think—really think—about what you're about to do. Don't ever do things quickly or without asking the Lord for His opinion. He wants you to have a sharp mind and stay focused on the task at hand. He desires the best for you, from the top of your head to the bottom of your toes. Filling up on fried or sugary foods won't just affect your waistline, it will also dull your senses and make you sluggish. For a sharper mind, make better choices.

Play a board game with a friend or loved one.

Trusting God

Lord, I ask You to renew my mind today. Keep thoughts of You front and center and help me to remain focused. Give me wisdom to know what to do to maintain clarity of thought for the journey ahead. Amen.

Today's Food Choices

(List all the foods you've eaten today)

_____

_____

_____

_____

Thoughts on Paper (Daily Journal Entry)

_____

_____

_____

_____

_____

_____

_____

_____

Metabolism

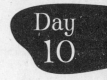

Tickler

Inside some of us is a thin person struggling to get out,
but he can usually be sedated with a few pieces of chocolate cake.
Author Unknown

Tidbit
Did You Know?

There is a difference between weight loss and burning fat. To lose
weight means to lose water and muscle tissue with little to no fat loss.
Burning fat means to lose fat tissue with no loss of water or muscle
tissue.[41]

············ (Trap) ··············

Comparing our size and shape with others.

We must be careful to remember that God deliberately created us different from one another. He didn't want us to be
clones. We are unique and special. Don't compare yourself
to a friend or family member. You are different for a reason.

Trick
Finish eating dinner before 7:00 p.m. so that you do not go to sleep
so soon after eating. Your body doesn't want to relax when it's still
processing food, so leave plenty of time for the "processing" before
bedtime.

Testimony

We all lose differently, don't we? Why is it that men can lose weight so fast? They just give up donuts for a few days, and they lose twenty pounds, just like that! A mere glance at a donut starts my hips to expand. It has taken me more than a couple of months to lose twenty pounds. And I had to give up a lot more than donuts to do it.

Gina Bishop

Treasure

In all these things we are more than conquerors through him who loved us.
ROMANS 8:37

Thought for the Day

We all have differing metabolisms. Some of us seem to run on high speed, others chug-chug along, practically on neutral. For some, losing weight seems to be a no-big-deal process. When they need to take off five or ten pounds, it seems to fall right off. Others can't seem to lose a pound, no matter how hard they try. Metabolism is a tricky thing. If you're on a low-calorie program, for example, you must determine how many calories a day your body is currently burning before you can determine how many you should be eating to lose weight. Using the formula of 3,500 calories = one pound, you can lose a pound a week if you cut back by 3,500 calories in that week. For example, if your body burns 2,100 calories a day (your current intake), and you cut back by 500 calories a day (dropping your daily intake to 1,600), it should result in a weight loss of about a pound a week. However, your metabolism also comes into play. Some people need more calories than others. Others can get by with less (but never less than 1,200 per day). It's a guessing game to get the numbers right, but the payoff is well worth the effort.

Trusting God

Father, I trust that You knew what You were doing when You created me. You designed this body of mine according to Your plan. Help me to see what I can do to keep my metabolism running smoothly. Help me to overcome my sluggish moments and give me energy from on high. Amen.

Today's Food Choices

(List all the foods you've eaten today)

_____

_____

_____

_____

Thoughts on Paper (Daily Journal Entry)

_____

_____

_____

_____

_____

_____

_____

Pollyanna Faith

Tickler

I never worry about diets.
The only carrots that interest me are
the number you get in a diamond.
Mae West

Tidbit
Did You Know?

A new indicator of child well-being shows that most children and adolescents have a diet that is poor or needs improvement, and that as children get older the quality of their diet declines.[42]

Trap

Salad dressings.

We love salads, in part because of the dressing we pour on top. We can load a salad with lots of healthy ingredients but then cover it with a high-calorie, high-fat, high-carb dressing. Before you use too much of your "dressing of choice," spend a little time researching the nutritional information. You might find a healthier alternative, such as lemon juice or a low-calorie/low-fat dressing.

Trick
Cut back strategically. This is such a simple concept that we often overlook it. If you're addicted to a particular food, don't attempt to stop eating it altogether. Instead, cut down with a clear strategy in

mind. Make a chart and stick with it. Instead of eating one cup of ice cream after dinner, measure out two-thirds of a cup. Over time, decrease the amount to half a cup.

Treat

Discover a new treat by perusing your local supermarket for exciting new snack ideas. Try something you've never before tried.

Testimony

Seems we churchgoers can't have a social without lots of food. Before and after Sunday school, the food tempts us. My stepmother called us the "meet and eat" folks. I've learned to grab a cup of tea and go talk with people. Doesn't always work, but most of the time it does. When I'm taking food to a social event, I always prepare a really healthy dish that I know I can eat without a problem, and I'll also make a sugar-free dessert. That way I can enjoy the social and feel good about what I'm eating.

Martha Rogers

Treasure

*And without faith it is impossible to please God,
because anyone who comes to him
must believe that he exists
and that he rewards those who earnestly seek him.*
HEBREWS 11:6

Thought for the Day

Pollyanna had an infectious optimism. Not a bad thing if it's rooted in real faith and hope. But sometimes in the real world it's hard to maintain optimism, particularly if it's a false optimism or one grounded in self. Acknowledging your struggles, dealing with them head-on, is a more practical way to overcome them. Plastering a false smile on your face, pretending everything is terrific, might make you look better, but it will ultimately leave you isolated. Let your optimism be rooted in the reality of God's overcoming power. Only then will it be truly infectious.

Turning Your Focus

Bake something special for a neighbor, friend, or shut-in.

Trusting God

Lord, I want to be optimistic, but I need to make sure my positive attitude is rooted in the right kind of faith, not in my own strengths. May I always recognize that every good thing comes from You, including all my accomplishments along the way. Amen.

Today's Food Choices
(List all the foods you've eaten today)

_____

_____

_____

_____

_____

_____

Thoughts on Paper (Daily Journal Entry)

_____

_____

_____

_____

_____

_____

_____

_____

_____

_____

_____

_____

_____

_____

_____

_____

_____

_____

_____

Pride Issues

Tickler

I don't want to draw too much attention to myself by being thin.
Anonymous

Tidbit
Did You Know?

"Because of intense demands for thinness, some people are at high risk for eating disorders—wrestlers, jockeys, cheerleaders, sorority members, socialites, dancers, gymnasts, runners, models, actresses, [and] entertainers."[43]

Trap

Taking a "day off" from your plan.

This might sound good in theory. After all, some would argue, we all need a "Sabbath rest" from our labors. However, a consistent plan of action is probably more practical in the long run. Sometimes, a day off can lead to two or three more—or even a dozen.

Trick
"Don't weigh your self-esteem. It's what's inside that counts."[44]

Veggies left unpeeled in the refrigerator probably won't be eaten. When you make your purchases, go ahead and peel them, placing them in airtight containers in the fridge. Try combining your favorite raw veggies, keeping a low-fat dressing nearby.

Testimony

To say I have a distorted body image is an understatement. When I'm Fat Marcia, I plod into a crowded room feeling like the biggest thing in there, convinced I'm taking up all available space. I fear that every eye is on me because I'm so obese. Conversely, when I lose a little weight, Foxy Marcia is unleashed and I glide into the room convinced that every eye is on me because I look so good. My husband says I think the world sets their watches to be up in time to look at me. I sure would like to find some middle ground.

Marcia Gruver

Treasure

Do not give the devil a foothold.
Ephesians 4:27

Thought for the Day

Pride rears its ugly head in ways that might surprise you. More often than not, we recognize pride when we focus on our own strengths. However, focusing on our weaknesses is also a form of pride. Anything that places our eyes on ourselves could be interpreted as pride. If you're struggling with self-image (i.e., having trouble seeing yourself the way God sees you), ask God to help you deal with the root of that problem: pride. If you're overly proud of "your" accomplishments, ask the Lord for a reality check. Leaning too far in either direction can be dangerous.

If you have a child in school,
choose a teacher and write him or her an encouraging note.

Trusting God

Lord, I ask You to deal with this pride of mine. Search me and know my heart today, Father. See if there is any root of pride in my life, whether insecurity or false security. Help me to lay down anything in my life that doesn't honor You. Amen.

Today's Food Choices

(List all the foods you've eaten today)

_____

_____

_____

_____

Thoughts on Paper (Daily Journal Entry)

_____

_____

_____

_____

_____

_____

Diversions

Tickler
*I bought a talking refrigerator that said
"Oink" every time I opened the door.
It made me hungry for pork chops.*
Marie Mott

Tidbit
Did You Know?

In 2000, annual U.S. vending machine sales were $36 billion.

In 2000, U.S. gumball sales were $500 million.[45]

····················(Trap)··················

Chips.

Many people have a hard time giving up chips (potato, corn, or otherwise). These tasty treats are nearly devoid of nutrition, yet are high in fat and salt. They're also addictive. Ever wonder why they advertise "you can't eat just one"? If you must have chips, reach for the baked variety and only purchase them in individual portion-controlled bags.

Trick

Only eat half of your dessert. If you must have a sweet treat after your meal, share it with a friend or split it in half, saving the second part for tomorrow.

Treat

Struggling with hunger late at night? Try a warm cup of bouillon.

Testimony

I thought I had the most kind, considerate, and generous boyfriend. But when I told him I wanted to go on a diet and exercise program, he had expensive candy sent to my office, and brought fresh pizzas to my door, again and again sabotaging my healthy efforts. He said I was fine the way I was—I who was more than one hundred pounds overweight. I actually believed him for a time, until I finally realized he wasn't kind and considerate to me at all. Soon I didn't have a boyfriend, and I finally realized that God wanted me to feel better about myself. And losing weight was one of the steps to feeling better.

Gina Bishop

Treasure

So then, let us not be like others,
who are asleep, but let us be alert and self-controlled.
1 THESSALONIANS 5:6

Thought for the Day

Some of our dieting diversions are simply poor habits, acquired over years of eating incorrectly. We sit down to watch a movie and feel cheated if we don't shovel down a bucket of popcorn. We finish a good meal and pout if we don't get a sugary dessert. We go out to eat at a buffet and fill our plate several times over, claiming we need to get our money's worth. Our needs aren't really needs at all. They are diversions. Many are simply amusements to which we have grown accustomed. However, we can gradually adopt new pastimes by making simple replacements. Our diversions themselves can be diverted.

······················(Turning Your Focus)··············

Buy a special treat for your pet or your friend's pet.

Trusting God

Lord, I ask for forgiveness for the many food-related "pets" I have acquired over the years. Reveal them all to me, Father. Help me to replace them with better choices. Give me the wisdom to know the difference. Amen.

Today's Food Choices
(List all the foods you've eaten today)

_____

_____

_____

_____

Thoughts on Paper (Daily Journal Entry)

Substitutions

Tickler

When I buy cookies, I eat just four and throw the rest away.
But first I spray them with Raid so I won't dig them out
of the garbage later. Be careful, though,
because that Raid really doesn't taste that bad.
Janette Barber

Tidbit
Did You Know?

There are more than 300,000 fast food restaurants in the United States.[46]

···················(Trap)··················

Diet sodas.

Many people drink diet drinks instead of drinking water, which would be far healthier and more satisfying. Diet drinks, especially those loaded with caffeine, can increase your appetite and leave you feeling thirstier than ever. Diet sodas might be handy, but they lack nutritional content, and in the long run they can be costly. Be sure to balance your soft drink intake with plenty of water.

Trick

Read nutrition labels. There's nothing like coming face-to-face with the calorie, fat, and carbohydrate content of your favorite candy bar.

························(Treat)······················

Struggling with a sweet tooth at mealtime? Try a baked sweet potato topped with butter spray (the no-calorie kind), a teaspoon of brown sugar, and one large marshmallow.

Testimony

My problem is that I love sweets, and one struggle I had with my diet was sugar highs and lows. But when I started baking with Splenda, I didn't notice a fluctuation of energy. The rollercoaster ride of sugar ups and downs was gone. Now I even sweeten my beverages with Splenda or Stevia (a natural herbal sweetener). Again, no ups and downs. Without the sugary highs and lows, my cravings for sweet foods have subsided.

Sharen Watson

Treasure

And the Lord said,
"Who then is that faithful and wise steward,
whom his master will make ruler over his household,
to give them their portion of food in due season?"
LUKE 12:42 NKJV

Thought for the Day

Sometimes even our substitutions can provide unnecessary temptation. Some people who would never consider consuming a regular
soft drink find themselves drinking six to eight diet sodas a day.
Others who would never eat a greasy hamburger will gobble down
three or four "diet" candy bars a day. The truth is, temptations are
temptations, regardless of the packaging. Too much of anything, even
something that seems good, can actually become a problem.

Turning Your Focus

Does your loved one have a favorite movie?
Consider purchasing it on VHS or DVD.

Trusting God

Father, I have to acknowledge that I still battle temptation. Help me to
recognize my weaknesses and avoid those things that seem to pull me
away from Your plan for my health. Amen.

Today's Food Choices

(List all the foods you've eaten today)

_____

_____

_____

_____

Thoughts on Paper (Daily Journal Entry)

Arguing with the Stomach

Tickler
*Each day, I try to enjoy something
from each of the four food groups:
the bonbon group, the salty snack group,
the caffeine group, and the
whatever-the-thing-in-the-tinfoil-in-the-back-of-the-fridge-is group.*
Unknown

Tidbit
Did You Know?

"Hunger is a signal telling the body that it needs to eat. It is also a signal to the body that it is in danger, that it needs food now. Our self-preservation instincts make us scarf down everything in sight in response to feelings of starvation. Our body doesn't care that we live in the modern world where food is plentiful. It acts the same as it would if we were living in the wild, having to hunt for our food."[47]

(Trap)

Hunger pangs.

We often eat the moment we experience hunger pangs. However, if we would pace ourselves, we would find that the pangs subside with time, especially if squelched with a large glass of water.

Trick

Stop eating when you are satisfied, not full.

Phoenix Hanna

(Treat)

Flavored rice cakes are filling and low in calories. Once consumed, they seem to swell, filling up that empty space and making you feel full.

Testimony

I heard a diet tip the other day. It was from a thin person, so I know it works. She told me to put my usual portion on the plate, and then remove one-fourth of it and throw it away. What a great idea. So, I'm thinking, "Does she mean one-fourth of every plateful?" It seemed like a simple concept. Just eat three sandwiches instead of four. I'm determined to try it, but I dread telling my stomach. You see, I've lost control—a problem that coincided with the growing popularity of all-you-can-eat buffets. I hope the method works for me as well as it worked for her. Because at least for now, the stomach rules.

Marcia Gruver

Treasure

*The sluggard's craving will be the death of him,
because his hands refuse to work.
All day long he craves for more.*
PROVERBS 21:25–26

Thought for the Day

Hunger pangs are tough to argue with. We convince ourselves (our minds, anyway), that we're going to do well today. Then the stomach intervenes, convincing us we're starving. Truthfully, we're anything but starving. Unfortunately, we don't usually wait out the first pangs of hunger. We give in to them. Time is the answer to this problem. Many of our hunger pangs are false, resulting from low blood sugar or a host of other problems. To give in to them too quickly—and with the wrong foods—can often worsen the problem. When it comes to arguing with the stomach, patience is the key. The next time that hunger strikes, slowly drink a large glass of water. Force yourself not to eat right away. Train yourself to say no to the initial pangs of hunger. If you can stave off that first attack, you could very well wait until your body is truly hungry to eat.

Turning Your Focus

Does your church put out a monthly newsletter?
Consider helping with the mailing process.

Trusting God

Lord, I confess that I often give in to my rumbling stomach and eat too much, too fast. Help me to train myself to wait on true hunger and to eat only the foods that will truly satisfy. Amen.

Today's Food Choices

(List all the foods you've eaten today)

_____

_____

_____

_____

Thoughts on Paper (Daily Journal Entry)

The Wall

Tickler
*I've been on a diet for two weeks
and all I've lost is fourteen days.*
Totie Fields

Tidbit
Did You Know?

More than 60 percent of adults do not achieve the recommended
amount of regular physical activity. In fact, 25 percent of adults
are not active at all. Inactivity increases with age, and it is more
common among women than men, and among those with lower
incomes and less education than among those with higher incomes
or education.[48]

Trap

Overconfidence.

If you place too much hope in your weight loss, you might
find yourself stunned when you hit a roadblock. You need to
be mentally prepared for obstacles so that they don't stop you
in your tracks.

Trick
Get a good night's sleep. You'll be able to make wiser choices if
you're fully awake and feeling good.

Testimony

I hit my first major roadblock after dropping forty pounds. It really scared me, because I still had a hundred pounds to go. I had grown overconfident somewhere along the way. I didn't waver from my plan—though I wondered for a couple of weeks if I'd ever lose any more weight. I picked up the pace on my exercise regimen and eventually the pounds started coming off again.

Janice Thompson

Treasure

Put no confidence in the flesh.
PHILIPPIANS 3:3

Thought for the Day

Walls are hard to climb—and even harder to knock down. They loom over us, casting frightening shadows. Though they seem like permanent roadblocks, they're really just diversions. It is possible to kick through them, stepping out into the sunshine on the other side. However, breaking through often requires an increase in exercise and stamina, so prepare yourself for more physical involvement.

Trusting God

Lord, when I hit those walls, remind me that they're not insurmountable. Help me see them for what they are—diversions. Give me the strength to break through them and continue on this road You've set before me. Amen.

Today's Food Choices

(List all the foods you've eaten today)

_____

_____

_____

_____

Thoughts on Paper (Daily Journal Entry)

_____

_____

_____

_____

_____

_____

_____

Falling Off the Wagon

Tickler

I go up and down the scale so often
that if they ever perform an autopsy on me
they'll find me like a strip of bacon —
a streak of lean and a streak of fat.
Texas Guinan

Tidbit

Did You Know?

Americans eat out an average of four to five times per week and spend approximately fifty cents of every food dollar outside the home.[49]

····························(Trap)··························

Equating a fall with permanent failure.

There's nothing like a tumble off the wagon to make us think we've "blown the diet for good." Nonsense. A tumble is just a tumble. Nothing permanent about it.

Trick

One thing that works for me is to brush my teeth immediately after supper. Then if my husband asks if I want a bowl of ice cream, I can say, "No, thanks, I've already brushed my teeth."
Rose McCauley

Testimony

It was a dark and stormy night, and the last thing I wanted to do was go home and eat my carefully planned, good-for-me diet dinner. Nothing would do except super-sized drive-thru food, the biggest dieting nemesis I have. I rushed home with my processed, hot-fried happiness-in-a-bag, polishing off thousands of calories in record time, giddy with how wonderful everything tasted.

The euphoria lasted for about an hour, at which time I became convinced I had consumed boulder-sized rocks. Not only had I fallen off the wagon, but I was too weak to get back on it for at least a couple days, having to be satisfied with the most bland foods in the universe. Since then, drive-thrus and I have had to part ways—hopefully forever.

Gina Bishop

Treasure

Then Jesus said to his disciples,
"If anyone would come after me,
he must deny himself and take up
his cross and follow me."
MATTHEW 16:24

Thought for the Day

Falling off the wagon is one thing; throwing in the towel is another thing altogether. We have to see our momentary lapses as what they are—momentary. We must stop believing they have permanent power over us. Today is today. Tomorrow is tomorrow.

Trusting God

Lord, help me to remove the words "I give up!" from my vocabulary. You never gave up on me, Father, and I shouldn't give up on myself, either. When I fail, and I know I will, please lift my eyes to You and give me hope for a new day. Amen.

Today's Food Choices

(List all the foods you've eaten today)

_____

_____

_____

_____

Thoughts on Paper (Daily Journal Entry)

_____

_____

_____

_____

_____

_____

_____

On the Rebound

Tickler

*I have gained and lost the same
ten pounds so many times,
over and over again,
that my cellulite must have déjà vu.*
Jane Wagner

Tidbit
Did You Know?

Although the American Heart Association recommends limiting fat to less than 30 percent of daily calories, most Americans get more than 40 percent of their daily calories from fat. Instead, you should limit the fat you consume to fifty to eighty grams per day.[50]

Trap

Seasons of celebration (holidays, weddings, birthdays, etc.).

We find it particularly difficult to rebound from holiday splurges, in part because we tend to lose sight of our goals when faced with a barrage of tempting goodies and celebrating family members. But there is truly no better time to bounce back than after a season of holiday feasting.

Trick

Plan ahead. For lack of a plan, would-be healthy eaters often find themselves cruising through fast-food restaurants on the way home from work. Plan a week's menus, and then make your shopping purchases accordingly. If necessary, prepare food in advance and freeze it.

Treat

Fruit and cheese kabobs. Using wooden skewers, combine chunks of your favorite fruits with cubes of low-fat cheese. These original treats are colorful, flavorful, and low in fat and calories.

Testimony

So what if you've failed along the way? So what if you had a sugar rush to lift you up? Done. Over. Move on. You are not perfect. You will never be perfect. So if all you did was eat a bowl of ice cream, well. . .no cows were killed in the making of this moment.

Kristin Billerbeck

Treasure

Consider it pure joy, my brothers,
whenever you face trials of many kinds,
because you know that the testing of your faith
develops perseverance.
JAMES 1:2–3

Thought for the Day

Keep the *re* in your plan! The prefix *re* means *to do again*. Get used to this prefix when trying to get in shape. Over and over again we stumble. Over and over we pick ourselves up, brush off the dust, and *re*bound into a new season. Isn't it terrific that the Lord allows us so many do-overs? He's such a generous and forgiving God. But we have to remember to forgive ourselves, as well. If we remove the *re* from our vocabulary, we stand to fail, for only in *re*inventing, *re*energizing, and *re*igniting the flame can we gain the courage and momentum to keep going.

Turning Your Focus

Purchase and read a book that's unlike
anything you've read before
(within reason, of course).

Trusting God

Lord, renew my mind today. Remind me that, even when I fall, You're here to pick me up. Amen.

Today's Food Choices

(List all the foods you've eaten today)

_____

_____

_____

_____

Thoughts on Paper (Daily Journal Entry)

_____

_____

_____

_____

_____

_____

_____

_____

_____

_____

_____

_____

_____

_____

_____

_____

_____

_____

Cheating Fairly

Tickler

Eat as much as you like.
Just don't swallow it.
Steve Burns

Tidbit
Did You Know?

Cabbage is 91 percent water.[51]

(**Trap**)

Nibbling while cooking.

Just a bite here, a tidbit there, and we've eaten half the meal before it ever lands on our plate. Develop a "no touch, no taste" policy. If you absolutely must taste test, only take a tiny bite or find a willing spouse or child for the job.

Trick
Don't skip meals. Doing so will make you ravenously hungry at the next meal, and you may find yourself gorging.

·· (Treat) ················

Sugar-free Jell-O. This delicious stuff comes in a variety of
flavors. It's colorful, fun, and tastes great. It's also deliciously
low in calories. Combine it with a bit of low-fat whipped
topping or a little fruit and you've got a tasty dessert with no
strings attached!

Testimony

Butter is such a delicious thing, but I end up wearing it on my hips if I'm not careful. So I use Butter Buds and get the nonfat butter spray. My popcorn and potatoes are properly dressed, and I'm less likely to head for the margarine container. Thank God for the advances in food sciences; processed foods can be a curse, but finding healthy alter-natives to artery-clogging foods is a definite blessing.

Lynette Sowell

Treasure

A wise man keeps himself under control.
PROVERBS 29:11

Thought for the Day

Is it okay to cheat on the road to good health? Of course. If we didn't ever give in, we would probably eventually snap and eat a full bag of cookies or a half-gallon of ice cream. If you must have a cookie, buy an individual package. Eat a couple and set the rest aside for another day. Measure out a half cup of your favorite ice cream and eat it slowly, letting it slowly dissolve—bit by tasty bit—on your tongue. This will go a long way toward satisfying those cravings, and you won't have to feel guilty afterward. You will have cheated fairly.

Cook a loved one's favorite meal.

Trusting God

Lord, I pray that You would bring a sense of balance into my life, especially when it comes to what I eat. Help me not to be too hard on myself, and to face each new day as a journey of its own.

Today's Food Choices

(List all the foods you've eaten today)

_____

_____

_____

_____

Thoughts on Paper (Daily Journal Entry)

_____

_____

_____

_____

_____

_____

_____

_____

20 Trust & Obey

Tickler
If you wish to grow thinner, diminish your dinner.
H. S. Leigh

Tidbit
Did You Know?

Americans aren't eating adequate amounts of the necessary vitamins and minerals—due, in part, to the consumption of junk food. According to a report in the American Journal of Clinical Nutrition, 31 percent of total calories in the average American's diet comes from snack foods, alcohol, and condiments that are not nutrient-dense.[52]

Trap

Putting too much trust in your "plan" and leaving God out of the equation.

Sometimes we do get a little heady about our plan of action, preaching its benefits to all who will listen. Instead, we should place our trust in God. After all, He was here long before humans concocted "the plan."

Trick
Don't turn back! "If you lose weight and then revert to your previous eating habits, you will also revert back to your previous weight. You have to take responsibility for the food you eat."
Janice LaQuiere

Testimony

There is food, glorious food, in my office practically every day of the week. There's always some meeting, seminar, or celebration that involves huge amounts of donuts, pizza, chips, and cake. I used to pretend to take just a small sample of the least offensive food and promise myself I wouldn't come back. But I always did, again and again. Now I re-route myself away from whatever part of the office is food friendly for that particular day. Sometimes I even leave the office at lunchtime to escape serious problems such as overwhelming pizza smells. Intense foods require drastic measures.

Gina Bishop

Treasure

Who among you fears the LORD
and obeys the word of his servant?
Let him who walks in the dark, who has no light,
trust in the name of the LORD and rely on his God.
ISAIAH 50:10

Thought for the Day

Is it easy to obey? Only when we truly relinquish all control and trust God completely. We can obey someone we trust, and our very loving and forgiving God has proven Himself trustworthy. He has our best interests at heart, so our obedience can be solidified in that hope. We will fall occasionally, but He is gracious to pick us back up, brush us off, and set us back on course. Obeying a God like that should be a piece of cake (pardon the pun).

Telephone someone from your church
you've been thinking of or missing.

Trusting God

Lord, I have to confess that obedience isn't always easy. Neither is
trusting. Please forgive me for the struggles I've had in this area and
remind me that, because I can trust You, my obedience should come
naturally. Amen.

Today's Food Choices

(List all the foods you've eaten today)

_____

_____

_____

_____

Thoughts on Paper (Daily Journal Entry)

_____

_____

_____

_____

_____

_____

_____

Fighting Off the Naysayers

Tickler

Thou shalt not weigh more than thy refrigerator.
Unknown

Tidbit
Did You Know?

The first step in dealing with diet sabotage. . .is to recognize it. Your saboteur may want to guard the status quo, keep you under control, or prevent your leaving to find a new life with your new body.[54]

(Trap)

Listening to others.

Sometimes we place too much stock in what other people say. Just a word can crush us. Or tempt us. Or send us off in a different direction. We need to stay focused on what God says about us, not what other people say.

Trick
Think about all the things you could do with the time and energy you spend worrying about your body and appearance. Try one.[55]

Salsa instead of mayo. This is a fun little trick. Try stirring a dollop of salsa into your tuna instead of the usual mayonnaise. Not only will you save calories, you will add a blast of unexpected flavor. Chances are you'll never go back to your old way of eating tuna again.

Testimony

During a call I made to an auto dealership, the tactful, well-bred salesman said to me, "Oh, I remember you. You're that little round girl." I decided on the spot that I was on a diet. At the time, I lived with my recently widowed mother, who was suffering from an extreme case of empty-nest syndrome. I returned to her house after work that night, whereupon she proudly placed a platter of crispy fried chicken in front of me. "I can't eat that," I said. "Why?" she countered. "Because I'm round," I sobbed. "I don't have anybody to cook for anymore," she wailed. I picked up a crunchy leg and tore into it. We sat across the table crying and eating chicken together.

Marcia Gruver

Treasure

*But the fruit of the Spirit is
love, joy, peace, patience, kindness, goodness,
faithfulness, gentleness and self-control.
Against such things there is no law.*
GALATIANS 5:22–23

Thought for the Day

Nothing can bring us down quicker than a negative word from a loved one, friend, or foe. There is such power in words. We let them stop us in our tracks, or even veer us off track. We let someone else's story of discouragement place an umbrella of despair over our own situation, when the two things are really unrelated.

The next time someone comes to you to bring you down about your plan of action, your past mistakes, or your so-called failings, remind yourself of who you are in Christ. Let their harsh words (which are often rooted in their own insecurities) roll off of you. Don't give them too much credence. God knows who you've been, who you are now, and who you are becoming. That's more than enough.

····················· (Turning Your Focus) ··············

Take a friend to the movies.

Trusting God

Lord, Yours is the only opinion that matters to me. May Your thoughts be my thoughts today and may I put the negative words of others where they belong—in the past, behind me. Amen.

Today's Food Choices

(List all the foods you've eaten today)

_____

_____

_____

_____

Thoughts on Paper (Daily Journal Entry)

_____

_____

_____

_____

_____

_____

_____

_____

_____

_____

_____

_____

_____

_____

_____

_____

_____

_____

_____

_____

_____

THE FINAL STRETCH

> You can't discover new lands
> without agreeing to lose sight of
> the shore for a very long time.
> ANONYMOUS

As the horses round the final stretch of the track, they catch a glimpse of the finish line. Sure, there are other horses closing in around them. They know that this last leg of the journey won't be easy. Nevertheless, they must persevere. They forge ahead, knowing that the next few moments of their lives could very well be the most important.

The same is true for you. You've faced some of your toughest challenges. You've tripped, fallen, and gotten back up again. You've run until your body is weary—and now, just about the time you think things are going to get easier, you have to gear up for the final stretch.

This last stage is usually the most deceptive, because people are in the habit of thinking, I'll just cut back until. . .until I reach my goal weight. . .until I have overcome poor eating habits. . .until I feel confident that I'll never revert to old ways again.

But here's the cold, hard truth: Watching your weight is a lifestyle. There is no finish line. Sure, you can focus on your "goal weight," but even that isn't really a stopping point. In fact, when you reach the desired goal, you have to fight to stay there.

How long?

For the rest of your life.

Yep. Just when you thought you could kick back, you discover what you've probably known all along but were too afraid to say.

In order to attain and maintain a healthy weight, you have to keep running.

Forever.

Enter the Zealot

Tickler
*All people are made alike—
of bones and flesh and dinner.
Only the dinners are different.*
Gertrude Louise Cheney

Tidbit
Did You Know?

The challenge for diet fanatics is to lose weight safely. Many diets don't just cut calories; they also limit foods that contain important nutrients that are essential for good health.[56]

Trap

Wearing out your family, friends, and coworkers.

Expecting others to behave as you behave and eat as you eat is a trap. Though you have learned some remarkable truths over the past few weeks, you cannot assume that others around you have been on the same learning curve. You must curb some of your enthusiasm and keep it in check so as not to overwhelm your family, friends, and coworkers.

Trick
Never talk about dieting when you're sharing a meal with friends. Others will feel more at ease and the focus will not be on you, which can prevent you from focusing on what "the other guy" is doing or saying.

Testimony

Everyone who loses a few pounds has a potential zealot living inside. In my case, I dropped the first ten or twenty pounds and the world began to take notice. As soon as they started asking the questions, I started giving the answers. I thought I had them all, because the weight was coming off so easily. Now, two years later, I'm struggling to maintain my weight loss and people are still asking questions. These days, my answers are a little slower in coming.

Janice Thompson

Treasure

*As you know,
we consider blessed those who have persevered.*
JAMES 5:11

Thought for the Day

When we first set out on the journey to lose weight, we do so with fear and trembling, feeling we know nothing about the process. At some point along the way, our confidence grows and we have a tendency to become self-proclaimed experts. Unfortunately, no one really gave us that title. We took it upon ourselves. And why not? We've come so far! We enjoy telling others about our journey. We don't even mind bragging a bit about the plan we've chosen. We purse our lips and shake our heads when we hear how others are losing weight. We offer advice freely. And we suggest that others follow our lead. Many of us transition from "I could care less" to "I'm putting everyone I know on a diet," and this can be very dangerous to friendships. In fact, many in our circle of influence might avoid us if we set out to "cure them" of their weight problems. Enthusiasm is one thing; fixing the world is quite another. We have to remember that God has given us one temple to care for. Just one.

Trusting God

God, I thank You for the energy and zeal You've given me to get into shape. I have needed the motivation every step of the way. Please help me not to go "over the top" when it comes to sharing my enthusiasm with others. Remind me that You haven't given other people to me like projects to be fixed. I have enough to do, keeping track of my own temple. Amen.

Today's Food Choices

(List all the foods you've eaten today)

_____

_____

_____

_____

Thoughts on Paper (Daily Journal Entry)

All Things in Moderation

Tickler
Your stomach shouldn't be a waist basket.
Author Unknown

Tidbit
"Check your thinking. You may be comparing yourself to others. . .
even your former self. Negative thinking will lead to a bad mood,
thereby increasing the risk of a lapse."[57]

> ## Trap
>
> Feeling deprived.
>
> The reason so many people can't stay with a healthy eat-
> ing plan is because they feel deprived. In order to avoid this
> feeling, you should occasionally have a moderate amount of
> something you crave. In fact, these tiny "cheats" will often
> keep you from falling off the wagon altogether.

Trick
Eat before you go to the grocery store. Don't ever go in with an empty
stomach, or your pocketbook and your health will both suffer the
consequences.

Testimony

By the time my son Chris approached his teens, it was a
stretch to say he was just chubby.
At age thirteen, his hormones
kicked in and he quickly became
enamored with an attractive
young girl at school. He went on
a diet to lose some of the weight,
not only adjusting his own eating habits, but also training his
parents on the foods they would
offer him. Through his self-discipline, he changed his eating
habits at home. However, he had
to devise a scheme to cope with
restaurant foods. He figured out
that eating less even when eating
out was an effective means for
weight control. Upon receiving
his food at a restaurant, he would
take his knife and cut down the
middle of his plate dividing the
food in half. He ate one half and
left the other half to either be
returned to the kitchen or taken
home. Through the years, he has
never faltered on the eating habits he established at age thirteen,
nor has he ever been overweight
from the time of his original
weight loss.

Frank A. Calzone

Treasure

Let your moderation be known unto all men.
The Lord is at hand.
PHILIPPIANS 4:5 KJV

Thought for the Day

You've heard the old expression, "You can't have your cake and eat it, too." Well, toss that idea. You can have your cake and you can eat it, just as long as you use a reasonable amount of common sense and portion control. A healthy lifestyle is all about balance. A full meal of celery sticks is no healthier than a plateful of chicken fried steak. Find a good middle ground, something you can live with, and stick with it. If you have trouble determining how much of a good thing you should allow yourself, try starting with half of whatever you're craving.

Turning Your Focus

Create a recipe file with your favorite new dishes.
Share the file with a friend.

Trusting God

Lord, I thank You for showing me how to live a life of moderation. The next time I'm faced with a challenge, help me to pass the test by controlling my urges. Curb my appetite, I pray, and show me how to stop when I've had enough. Amen.

Today's Food Choices

(List all the foods you've eaten today)

_____

_____

_____

_____

Thoughts on Paper (Daily Journal Entry)

Just a Spoonful of Sugar

Tickler
Forget love. . . I'd rather fall in chocolate!
Author Unknown

Tidbit
Did You Know?

"U.S. consumers spent more than $24.3 billion on candy in 2002, a 1.6 percent increase over 2001, according to figures based on the U.S. Department of Commerce 2002 Confectionary Report and issued by the National Confectioners Association. On average, consumers made $84.34 worth of candy purchases" in 2002, up 0.3 percent from the previous year.[59]

Trap

Sweet tea.

For those of us from the South, in particular, sweet tea can become a familiar old friend. Try substituting Splenda for sugar. If that doesn't satisfy you, then slowly (over a period of a week or so) start cutting back on the sugar until you've got it down to a minimal level.

Trick
Sometimes you should skip the chicken and eat the cookie. However, you can't eat both the chicken and the cookie.
Janice LaQuiere

Treat

Cinnamon toast. Start with a piece of low-cal or low-carb bread. Toast it and add zero-calorie spray butter, cinnamon, and Splenda (or low-cal sweetener of your choice).

Testimony

I like to tweak my diet plan now and then. By throwing in some different items to the same old diet routine, it helps in heading off cravings. I try exotic teas and coffees, fancy spices, and what I think is a real find—a huge jar of multicolored jimmies. They're cute, they're colorful, and just a shake or two makes the lowliest dessert. . .well, kind of fun.

Gina Bishop

Treasure

For God did not give us a spirit of timidity,
but a spirit of power, of love and of self-discipline.
2 TIMOTHY 1:7

Thought for the Day

For those who want an occasional sweet, a small amount of sugar is usually the way to go (except for diabetics, of course). If you overload your body with a large quantity of sugar, eventually you'll crash. However, just a small bit of sweetness—say one cookie, as opposed to five or six—is certainly the way to curb your craving without crashing afterward. Sugar in large quantities can lead to a host of health-related problems, but just a spoonful now and then won't do much damage.

····· (Turning Your Focus) ··············

Instead of eating that sweet yourself,
give it away to someone special.

Trusting God

Lord, I thank You that I don't have to have a huge amount of anything. Tiny nibbles are enough, especially when it comes to sweets. Guard my heart in this area, Father. Amen.

Today's Food Choices

(List all the foods you've eaten today)

_____

_____

_____

_____

Thoughts on Paper (Daily Journal Entry)

_____

_____

_____

_____

_____

_____

_____

_____

Buffet Line Woes

Tickler
We never repent of having eaten too little.
Thomas Jefferson

Tidbit
Did You Know?

With our juggled lifestyles, dining out has taken on an important role in the average American household. One in every three people eats away from home at any one mealtime. It is possible to dine out, in various settings, and still eat healthfully—it just takes some planning.[60]

····················(Trap)··················

Eating when full.

We used to call it the "clean your plate club" when I was a kid. The problem with cleaning your plate is that you're often full before the food is gone. Let's create a new club and call it the "ditch the leftovers" club. We'll be a lot healthier and the dues aren't nearly as high.

Trick
Portion control is the key, especially when you're eating out. If you find yourself in a tempting buffet line, take teeny-tiny spoonfuls of "the good stuff" and moderately larger portions of the healthy stuff.

The next time you're at a buffet, gravitate toward the fruit, salad, and vegetables. More and more restaurants are including these healthy items on their buffet, and why not? You might be surprised to find items just as tasty (if not more so) than the high-calorie, high-fat choices.

Testimony

After not feeling well drove me to much prayer, God revealed that I ate too many sweets, fats, and spicy foods, and that my portion sizes resembled Pikes Peak. My husband took me to a Chinese restaurant with a wonderful buffet of tantalizing dishes that tempted me to ignore God's words. When nausea reared its ugly head, I determined to do well, and ordered a healthy-sounding dish from the menu: kung poa chicken. When the waiter brought my plate, my eyes widened in horror as I stared at an enormous meal laced with red-hot peppers. At first, I was disappointed when one bite exposed its spiciness, but then it dawned on me what a sense of humor my heavenly Father has, and to what extreme he would go to keep me from overeating. I giggled each time I took a bite of my small portion of rice and extremely bland egg drop soup.

Deb Ullrick

Treasure

Do not join those who drink too much wine
or gorge themselves on meat.
PROVERBS 23:20

Thought for the Day

Somehow our mentality changes when we go out to eat. Because we're paying directly for our food, we feel we must treat it differently. We must get our money's worth. And restaurants make it easy, offering huge portions and tantalizing us with appetizers and desserts. However, it is possible to eat out, even at a buffet, and still get your money's worth. After all, good health saves us money, too. If we pass up that second helping of egg foo yong, we might very well avoid a trip to the doctor's office or a run to the drugstore for antacids.

············ (Turning Your Focus) ··············

Plan a one-day vacation or outing with a loved one.

Trusting God

Lord, it's hard to be reasonable at a buffet. Sometimes I just get so caught up in the moment that I forget about the future. Help me to eat in moderation, Father, even when eating out. Amen.

Today's Food Choices

(List all the foods you've eaten today)

_____

_____

_____

_____

Thoughts on Paper (Daily Journal Entry)

Addicted No More

Tickler
If I can't have too many truffles, I'll do without.
Colette

Tidbit
Did You Know?

Caffeine can temporarily speedup your heart rate, wake you up, and give you a burst of energy, but the effects are short-term. To cut back on caffeine, the American Dietetic Association recommends that you start gradually to avoid withdrawal headaches.[61]

Trap

Refusing to admit you have an addiction.

Anyone who has attended a 12-step meeting knows that admitting the problem is half the battle. The same is true with food addictions. You must face them head-on, admitting that they are a problem. Only then will you be able to overcome them.

Trick
Take your salad dressing on the side. Then dip the prongs of your fork into it before each bite.

Testimony

I recently spoke to a man who shared that he had grown so addicted to caffeine that he couldn't function without it. Finally, under direct orders from the Lord, he gave it up. Whether you struggle with an addiction to sugar, caffeine, fried foods, or something else, the Lord doesn't want you to grow so attached to any particular thing that you can't do without it. He is an addiction-breaking God who wants to see us set free from every form of bondage.

Janice Thompson

Treasure

When the perishable has been clothed with the imperishable,
and the mortal with immortality,
then the saying that is written will come true:
"Death has been swallowed up in victory."
1 CORINTHIANS 15:54

Thought for the Day

Addictions begin in the mind and heart and gravitate to the stomach, don't they? We "want" something, and once we grow attached to it, we "need" it. Problem is, we never really needed it in the first place. Our bodies can grow chemically addicted to certain foods, particularly sweets and caffeine. Then, if we try to stop eating them, our bodies cry out in pain: "Feed me some of that! Now!" The best way to end an addiction is to taper back gradually. If your body is truly addicted, stopping caffeine and/or sugar immediately can lead to headaches and other problems. Set yourself up on a schedule to "ease your way out of" food addictions. Before long, both your mind and your body will thank you. The Lord truly wants to see you set free from addictions.

········· (Turning Your Focus) ·············

Consider helping out at your local 12-step program.

Trusting God

Lord, please help me overcome my food addictions. Show me what they are. Reveal truth to me. Then help me walk as an overcomer. I don't want to be addicted any longer, Father, but I need Your help. Amen.

Today's Food Choices

(List all the foods you've eaten today)

_____

_____

_____

_____

Thoughts on Paper (Daily Journal Entry)

Tickler

Obesity is really widespread.
Joseph O. Kern II

Tidbit

Did You Know?

In a study of nine-to-fifteen-year-old girls, slightly more than half reported use of exercise to lose weight, and slightly less than half ate less to lose weight. Approximately one in twenty reported using diet pills or laxatives to lose weight.[62]

Trap

Skipping breakfast.

Many of us were raised in homes where breakfast was overlooked. Unfortunately, as we've heard so many times, breakfast is the most important meal of the day. Did you know, for example, that people who eat breakfast actually lose more weight than those who choose to skip it? Start a new family trend and teach your children and grandchildren to eat a healthy breakfast.

Trick

Here's something you can teach your children. Leave space on your plate between foods so that none of them touch. You'll still get the effect of a full plate without all of the calories.

Treat

Here's a yummy treat you can pass down to your kids: "Ants on a log." Take a piece of celery, spread a tablespoon of low-fat peanut butter on it, and sprinkle a few raisins on top.

Testimony

As I was growing up, my mother always tried to encourage me to lose weight. However, she did not often give me the right kinds of food. We always ate breakfast, which was a good habit, but what we ate was gravy, biscuits, eggs, bacon, and other fried foods. I still remember that she would occasionally try to reduce my intake by limiting me to two biscuits. At least she taught me to limit myself, and as a result I find I have more will power to cut down my meals today. As an adult, when I want to lose weight, I try to cut my food portions in half—and it works. I also try to eat the right foods, not all fried or full of fat. Fat makes one fatter.

Charlotte Holt

Treasure

I will bring them back from captivity.
Ezekiel 29:14

Thought for the Day

In some families, weight is a primary issue. In some cases, parents force their children to look a certain way, guarding every morsel of food that goes into their mouths. Consequently, the children end up obsessed about their weight. In other cases, parents soothe their children's woes by feeding them—often too much or the wrong things. Many of these children grow into hefty adults, simply because of lack of training or balance. If you come from a family where the focus on food was skewed, there is hope. Regardless of your family background, you can start fresh—for your own well-being and also as a balanced model for your children and grandchildren to follow.

· · · · · · · · · · · · · (Turning Your Focus) · · · · · · · · · · · · ·

Invest in a child's life today.

Trusting God

Lord, I choose to lay aside all of the bad habits and personal issues concerning food from my past. Help me to start fresh today. Show me how to train up the next generation to eat right. Amen.

Today's Food Choices
(List all the foods you've eaten today)

_____

_____

_____

_____

Thoughts on Paper (Daily Journal Entry)

Feeding My Broken Heart

Tickler
"Stressed" spelled backwards is "desserts."
Coincidence? I think not!
Author Unknown

Tidbit
Did You Know?

A study reported in *Drugs and Therapy Perspectives* states that about 1 percent of women in the U.S. have a binge-eating disorder, as do 30 percent of women who seek treatment to lose weight. In other studies, up to 2 percent of American adults (1 to 2 million people) have problems with binge eating.[63]

Trap

"Loaded" ice creams.

Ice cream in and of itself probably wouldn't be terribly harmful. But today's ice creams are loaded with chunks of everything from candy bars to cookies. With every bite, we get more sugar and less cream. Be careful not to fall into the "loaded" ice cream trap, especially when you're feeling a little blue. The extra pounds will only make you bluer, after all.

Trick

Occasionally reward yourself for your new healthy lifestyle by purchasing a new clothing item. There's nothing like a new outfit to make you feel like a new person.

Treat

Next time you're feeling down, instead of reaching for something loaded with sugar, try exercise instead. Nothing will pull you out of the depths quicker than a brisk walk or some abdominal crunches.

Testimony

New clothes make you feel good. So what if it's not the size you want them to be? Get something slimming, and feel great. I bought new clothes for a recent event. They were expensive and were completely unnecessary for my lifestyle here in Auburn. (I even got Prada shoes off eBay). Well, you know, I felt like a chick. When a friend saw me, she said, "I thought your book signing was tomorrow, but when I saw you dressed like that, I knew I'd missed it!"

Kristin Billerbeck

Treasure

No one will offer food to comfort those
who mourn for the dead—
not even for a father or a mother—
nor will anyone give them a drink to console them.
JEREMIAH 16:7

Thought for the Day

Those who struggle with depression can attest to the fact that food can become closely linked to how we feel. When we feel great, we celebrate with food. When we get depressed, we feed ourselves to dull the pain. Unfortunately, putting on extra pounds only causes us to be more depressed, so we find ourselves in a vicious cycle. First of all, if you are facing a serious depression, it might be time to see a doctor. He can help you get back on the right track. There are a few "pick me ups" that really do help people who are struggling with mild depression. Take your eyes off yourself and do something for someone else today. Take an elderly neighbor for a drive or deliver a meal to a sick friend. Next, get some exercise. Exercise will often lift you out of the doldrums. Finally, be careful not to give in to the temptation to feed your sadness, particularly with sugars. God is standing by, ready to take your cares and sorrows. Give them to Him. Don't feed them.

Turning Your Focus

Follow the advice above and visit with
an elderly neighbor or a shut-in.

Trusting God

Lord, this is such a struggle in my life. Instead of giving problems over to You, I often feed them. Release me from this bondage today, Father. Lift me out of any depression and restore my hope. Amen.

Today's Food Choices

(List all the foods you've eaten today)

_____

_____

_____

_____

Thoughts on Paper (Daily Journal Entry)

Choices

Tickler
*In general, mankind, since the improvement of cookery,
eats twice as much as nature requires.*
Benjamin Franklin

Tidbit
Did You Know?

"In 2000, Americans spent $13 billion on chocolate in all its forms."[64]

······················(Trap)·····················

Trendy coffee shops.

Oh, how we love our coffee. We will pay almost any price
for a steaming cup of the stuff. Strong, sweet, flavored, loaded
with zing, we just can't seem to live without it. Take inventory
of where your coffee habits are. What exactly are you spend-
ing for a cup of your favorite brew and how many calories or
carbs does it contain? Can you taper back?

Trick
If you buy low-fat foods, like baked chips instead of the regular ones,
eat the same serving size as before. Don't double your portion just
because the chips are low-fat.
Phoenix Hanna

Testimony

I had been trying to lose a few pounds. On my usual Friday night run to the store, I grabbed a cart and started up and down the aisles, loading in my week's groceries. As I started up the snack aisle, where all the chips, crackers, cookies, and other goodies are located, I "heard" the following statement: "Make no provision for the flesh." I started laughing, said, "Yes, Lord," backed immediately out of that aisle, and hurried on to the next. I've never forgotten it. I learned two very important things from that experience: (1) God is interested in our health and well-being, and He truly watches over us every minute; and (2) His Word covers every situation of life.

Dorothy Clark

Treasure

Do not lie to each other,
since you have taken off your old self with its practices.
COLOSSIANS 3:9

Thought for the Day

When faced with choices, we often make the wrong ones. Sometimes, there seems to be a dizzying array of foods to pick from and we can't make up our minds. This is when careful advance preparation comes in handy. If you've already packed your lunch for work, you won't be as likely to "grab a bite to eat" with friends and coworkers. If you've already written down your plan for the day, you won't be as likely to grab a candy bar from the vending machine. Having choices isn't really a bad thing. Just be sure to make the right one when confronted with too many.

········· (Turning Your Focus) ··············

Give your spouse, child, or friend a greeting card.
Just because.

Trusting God

Lord, thanks for giving me choices. I know life would get pretty boring without them. Help me make the right ones today, Father—choices that will keep me healthy and strong. Amen.

Today's Food Choices

(List all the foods you've eaten today)

_____

_____

_____

_____

Thoughts on Paper (Daily Journal Entry)

_____

_____

_____

_____

_____

No More Excuses

Tickler
I'm not overweight.
I'm just nine inches too short.
Shelley Winters

Tidbit
Did You Know?

Some people actually "excuse" themselves from eating right all of their lives. Many even pass these excuses on to their children.

················· Trap ·················

Excusing ourselves.

Sometimes we have legitimate excuses for slipping. Other times we "come up with" excuses to validate our behavior. In many cases, we've been trained since childhood to act this way. It's time to put our excuses behind us and move forward into the future that God has for us.

Trick
Don't keep junk food in the house. That way, when you get stressed, you won't have a "stash" of goodies waiting.

Testimony

Sometimes I wonder if some of my eating patterns are hormonal. I'm forty-eight and sometimes around "that time of the month" I could eat the kitchen sink. I've also read that when you get close to the change of life, things that used to not bother you, do, and things that used to bother you, don't. That might explain some of my mood swings lately, but not all. I think I was coming under conviction for out-of-control eating; for giving food a place in my life that it was not meant to have. I'm hoping to start giving God that place.

Deb Ullrick

Treasure

But they all alike began to make excuses.
LUKE 14:18

Thought for the Day

Excuses, excuses, excuses. I can't eat right because I never seem to lose weight. I can't stick with a program because I have no willpower. I can't help it if I'm overweight—it runs in my family. I have to eat what my family eats. On and on the list goes. We often grow so accustomed to our list of excuses that we don't remember that the Lord can deliver us from them. Instead of excusing our poor behaviors, we need to confront them. If you're struggling with your willpower, give it over to the Lord. If you come from a family that didn't care about weight gain, then acknowledge that and learn from it. Don't ever give in to the excuses. Most likely, they are just misappropriated defenses for wrong behaviors. Let down your defenses today and see what the Lord can do.

····· · · · · · · · (Turning Your Focus) · · · · · · · · · · ·

Watch the sunset tonight,
possibly with a friend, loved one, or pet.

Trusting God

Lord, I know You're probably tired of all my excuses. I know I am.
Help me to admit the truth. Give me the courage to face real issues
head-on and show me Your way, Lord. Amen.

Today's Food Choices

(List all the foods you've eaten today)

_____

_____

_____

_____

Thoughts on Paper (Daily Journal Entry)

_____

_____

_____

_____

_____

_____

_____

_____

Living the Life

Tickler
I feel about airplanes the way I feel about diets.
It seems to me that they are wonderful things
for other people to go on.
Jean Kerr

Tidbit
Did You Know?

Twenty-five percent of American men and 45 percent of American women are on a diet on any given day.[66]

Trap

Temporary Fixes.

One of the best things people can remember is that a diet should not be thought of as something temporary. If you're going to make dietary changes, or activity changes, consider them as lifestyle changes. Consider them as things that are going to help you look better, feel better, lower your stress, improve your physical and mental performance, and allow you to enjoy life.[67]

Trick

Sign up for a dance class or purchase a how-to line-dancing video you can use in the privacy of your own home.

Treat

Exercise can be a treat! Are you searching for a fun way to exercise? Exercise balls can be incorporated into almost any fitness plan, including aerobics, bodybuilding, and weightlifting, among others.[69]

Testimony

I love to read, and I love to have my own books, but they can be expensive. I really enjoy going to the used bookstores, and once inside, I go straight to their clearance racks to pick up an armful of books for just a few dollars. I stay within my budget, I get to have my own books, and as I sink into my favorite easy chair, I've created a diverting time away from snacking and other food temptations.

Gina Bishop

Treasure

Everyone born of God overcomes the world.
This is the victory that has overcome the world,
even our faith.
1 JOHN 5:4

Thought for the Day

Life is all about living. Enjoying. Relishing in the small things. If we get too hung up on our weight or how we look, we can forget to live. We need to remember that God helps us overcome not just physically but also spiritually and emotionally. He is a victorious God and He wants us to triumph in this life, as well. Regardless of where you are in your journey toward good health, take some time to enjoy life today. Work in your garden, telephone a friend, write a letter, or take a walk. Visit with the Lord and thank Him for sharing His goodness with you.

Trusting God

Lord, I love You. I probably don't tell You often enough, but I do. And I'm so grateful You gave me life in the first place. You are an awesome God and I praise You for all You've done in me, through me, and around me. I bless You, Lord! Amen.

Today's Food Choices

(List all the foods you've eaten today)

_____

_____

_____

_____

Thoughts on Paper (Daily Journal Entry)

_____

_____

_____

_____

_____

_____

_____

Light-Hearted Living

Tickler

If you hang your swimsuit on the refrigerator door,
the goodies inside will be easier to ignore.
Author Unknown

Tidbit
Did You Know?

Laughter burns calories! "When we laugh, the rib muscles, the abdominal wall muscles, and the diaphragm all move as we let out a long breath of air ended by a 'ha' sound. The lungs then take in more oxygen as we breathe in deeply. Our heart rate increases, pumping blood and carrying oxygen to all the body cells. Endorphins, our natural pain killers, are released, so after laughing we feel a sense of relaxation."[69]

Trap

Heavy lunches. Sometimes we feel especially "heavy" in the afternoons because we've eaten a heavy lunch or snacked on sugary products in the midafternoon. To get through the afternoon without a slump, stay away from sweets and don't overload at mealtime.

Trick

Learn to laugh at yourself. Instead of moping over how you look, take a little time to have fun at your own expense. When you catch a glimpse of yourself in a window, instead of moaning over how you look, take a second glance and utter the words everyone loves to hear: "Who is that knockout?"

Treat

Figs. "Because they have no fat, saturated fat, cholesterol, or sodium, figs help you meet dietary guidelines established by the U.S. Department of Agriculture. Fig puree can be used to replace fat in baked goods."[70]

Testimony

Several years ago, just after I began First Place (a Christian weight-loss program), I made brownies for a party at church. Because I made several batches to take, I had leftovers and brought them home. All night I thought about those brownies and how good they'd taste. I'd gone without chocolate and sweets for so long. Then I decided I didn't need them and prayed for God to take away the desire. The next morning, I decided that one little bit wouldn't hurt. Well, when I opened them up to get one, they were covered with ants. I mean the ants were swarming over those brownies. God does have a sense of humor.

Martha Rogers

Treasure

"For my yoke is easy and my burden is light."
MATTHEW 11:30

Thought for the Day

Laughter is indeed good medicine. We've heard this all our lives, but how quickly we forget. We need to learn to kick back and not take everything so seriously. A good attitude isn't just good for your morale, it's great for your body, too. According to www.holistic-online. com: "Laughter brings in positive emotions that can enhance—not replace—conventional treatments. Hence it is another tool available to help fight disease. Experts believe that, when used as an adjunct to conventional care, laughter can reduce pain and aid the healing process. For one thing, laughter offers a powerful distraction from pain."[71]

· · · · · · · · · · · · · (**Turning Your Focus**) · · · · · · · · · · · · · ·

Take time today to read a couple of those
silly forwarded e-mails your friends keep sending you.

Trusting God

Thank You, Lord, for bringing joy into my life. You've replaced the pain with an abounding peace and I'm so thankful. You're such a gracious God, to give me such good gifts. Keep my heart "light" and my spirit full. Amen.

Today's Food Choices

(List all the foods you've eaten today)

_____

_____

_____

_____

Thoughts on Paper (Daily Journal Entry)

A Wrinkle in Time

Tickler

*Wrinkles should merely indicate
where smiles have been.*
Mark Twain

Tidbit
Did You Know?

"When you have a positive self-image, you value and respect your body. You are also more likely to feel good about living a healthy lifestyle."[72]

Trap

Forbidden Foods.

If you create a list (real or subconscious) of forbidden foods, you will be far more likely to crave those things. Remember that all foods are given by God for our enjoyment. It's just a matter of portion control.

Trick
Here's a tip that a very trim woman in her seventies passed on to me (though I haven't tried it yet): Whenever the scales go a couple of pounds above your target weight, just eat an apple for supper a couple of nights.
Rose McCauley

By substituting fish for chicken or beef two or three times a week, you'll avoid storing an excess 300 calories. Fish, available in many varieties, can be prepared in a jiffy and supplies omega-3 fatty acids, which are critical to proper cell function and healthy skin.[73]

Testimony

My son Chris implemented an exercise routine at the same time he initiated his diet. This included lifting weights, jogging, and riding his bike. These activities have also been maintained over the years. His jogging was inspired by his grandfather, who started jogging at the age of sixty-seven and competed in his last 10K race at the age of eighty-seven. I think it is safe to say that Grandpa also taught Chris the significance of dedication to a cause.

Frank A. Calzone

Treasure

Does the clay say to the potter,
"What are you making?"
ISAIAH 45:9

Thought for the Day

Our bodies almost seem to betray us as we grow older, don't they? Things that used to be firm are now soft, things that used to be "up" are now "down," and we don't seem to have any control over it. Part of the joy of celebrating the Lord's goodness in our lives is realizing that He made each of us unique and special. As we age, we will undergo changes, but if we embrace them and smile at each little discovery, chances are we'll develop a "God-image" of ourselves instead of a "self-image."

Trusting God

Lord, You knew what You were doing when You created me. I trust You with this body of mine, Father. I know it's not really mine—but Yours. Thank You for entrusting it to me. Amen.

Today's Food Choices

(List all the foods you've eaten today)

_____

_____

_____

_____

Thoughts on Paper (Daily Journal Entry)

_____

_____

_____

_____

_____

_____

_____

It's Not
How You Look

Tickler
The older you get, the harder it is to lose weight,
because by then your body and
your fat have become good friends.
Author Unknown

Tidbit
Did You Know?

"Eighty percent of American women are dissatisfied with their appearance."[74]

· (Trap) · · · · · · · · · · · · · · · ·

Fear of the mirror.

The mirror provides a reflection of our outward appearance, but it doesn't say anything about the inner person. Many of us avoid the mirror like the plague. But instead of cringing when you look in the mirror, spend a while contemplating the fact that you were created in God's image.

· ·

Trick
If you go out to eat, share your meal with a friend. You'll save money and calories.

Testimony

A funny aside to my weight-loss journey is what it means to be an overweight runner. Most runners are so thin that if they were chickens you wouldn't even be able to make a decent soup out of them. They are scrawny. I am not scrawny. Even when I am thin, I am large: size 11 feet, 7-inch wrists. (Thanks for those genes, Dad!) For a girl with a little meat on her bones, running can be a little more challenging. The seismic activity felt by neighboring communities would be troublesome.

Mary Hanlon

Treasure

*You stare and stare at the obvious,
but you can't see the forest for the trees.*
2 CORINTHIANS 10:7 THE MESSAGE

Thought for the Day

From the time we were children, we were judged by our appearance. As we grew, we learned to turn to magazine images, television, and movie stars to show us what we should look like. When we didn't measure up to their standards, depression would set in. Take heart! Other people may look at our outward appearance, but God looks at our hearts. It's His desire for us to be freed from the bondage of caring too much about what we look like. When you take a look in the mirror, look beyond the "trees" as the verse above suggests. Don't worry about how chubby your thighs look or the protrusion in your midsection. And when a few pounds come off, enjoy the new look—but don't place too much confidence in it. Instead, look at all of the amazing things the Lord has accomplished in your life and in the lives of those around you. There's so much to celebrate!

> ·············(Turning Your Focus)··············
> Take someone you love on a picnic.
> If you choose to go alone,
> take a good book along.
> Be sure to load your picnic basket with
> your favorite fruits and veggies.

Trusting God
Lord, please deliver me from caring too much about how I look. Take the air-brushed magazine images out of my head and give me a healthy image of how I should look, based solely on Your design for my life and body. Amen.

Today's Food Choices
(List all the foods you've eaten today)

_____

_____

_____

_____

Thoughts on Paper (Daily Journal Entry)

A Healthy Me

Tickler
Eat. . .to live, and do not live to eat.
William Penn

Tidbit
Did You Know?

"There is evidence to suggest that a high intake of fruit and vegetables decreases the risk of lung cancer."[76]

> **Trap**
>
> "I must stay fired up!"
>
> "To be motivated, you don't need to be fired up or excited. Those emotions won't sustain you over the long haul anyway. You just need the calm, certain conviction that you are ready for a real change."[77]

Trick
"Set a regular time and place to dine. Many of us associate eating with other activities, such as watching TV or going to the movies. Soon we find that activities like turning on the TV also turn on our desire to eat. Help your family break the habit of automatic eating by making one simple rule: Eat only while seated at the dining table."[77]

Testimony

I went for a checkup after losing one hundred pounds. When my doctor walked in the room, I saw that she was probably a good eighty pounds overweight. After examining me, she proclaimed that I was the healthiest woman she'd ever seen and asked me for my secret to weight loss. Go figure!

Janice Thompson

Treasure

Lord, by such things men live;
and my spirit finds life in them too.
You restored me to health and let me live.
ISAIAH 38:16

Thought for the Day

Our health is far more important than how we look. With all of the risks related to weight gain, we should celebrate every pound lost. Each step toward our goal is a step away from a life of chronic health problems. In my case, I waved good-bye to sleep apnea after losing the first fifty pounds. By the time I had dropped one hundred pounds, my cholesterol was normal and my blood pressure looked great. There's nothing better than feeling good to keep you motivated, unless perhaps it's a clean bill of health.

Consider taking a new friend to lunch.

Trusting God

Lord, I thank You for giving me victory over health problems. As I inch my way toward the goal, help me to be thankful for each small victory. Help me to complete the journey to great health so that I can better serve You. Amen.

Today's Food Choices

(List all the foods you've eaten today)

_____

_____

_____

_____

Thoughts on Paper (Daily Journal Entry)

_____

_____

_____

_____

_____

_____

_____

_____

Realistic Goals

Tickler
I'm allergic to food.
Every time I eat it breaks out into fat.
Jennifer Greene Duncan

Tidbit
Did You Know?

"Losing weight in a healthy way does not involve starving or deprivation. That's why it's permanent. If you lose weight in a healthy way, you're likely to keep it off for good."[79]

Trap

Eating late.

If you must eat at night, eat light. Going to bed on a full stomach can make it difficult to sleep, and it gives you less time to work off what you've eaten.

Trick
"Find a method of exercise that you enjoy and do it regularly. Don't exercise to lose weight or to fight your body. Do it to make your body healthy and strong and because it makes you feel good."[80]

Try mixing low-fat whipped cream and blueberries for a fluffy treat. Substitute strawberries, raspberries, or your berry of choice.

Testimony

A friend of mine was trying to help me get started to lose some weight. She suggested that I try her never-fail diet for two weeks, and she guaranteed I'd lose weight. I did, but it took every ounce of willpower to stick to it because it was boring: Half a grapefruit for breakfast, with water or tea. Salad with vinegar and oil dressing for lunch (with lots of goodies in the salad like celery, broccoli, etc.). No croutons or carrots—too fattening. Supper was a diet type of fish (not salmon or cod—too fattening). You could have as much squash, peas, or green beans as you liked with it. Great diet—I lost ten or twelve pounds—but afterward was the problem. How long can you go on eating salad, squash, and fish?

Sue Timm

Treasure

You were bought at a price.
Therefore honor God with your body.
1 Corinthians 6:20

Thought for the Day

If we've learned anything over the past several weeks, it's this: Weight loss shouldn't happen overnight. We must set realistic, practical goals—short term and long term. Then, when we fall, we need to brush ourselves off and continue as if nothing happened. Short-term goals give us hope. We can reach them, catch our breath, and move forward. Long-term goals give us something to work toward. Whether you've reached your long-term goal at this point or not, do not give up! Instead, just look how far you've come.

Trusting God

Lord, I thank You for showing me how to set goals. Remind me every day that I will not progress unless I set my sights on the prize. And thank You for giving me a glimpse of the prize on this journey. What a blessing! Amen.

Today's Food Choices

(List all the foods you've eaten today)

_____

_____

_____

_____

Thoughts on Paper (Daily Journal Entry)

_____

_____

_____

_____

_____

_____

_____

_____

Forever?

Tickler
A waist is a terrible thing to mind.
Tom Wilson

Tidbit
Did You Know?

"After you've gained some familiarity with your body's cues, it will be clear to you when you're experiencing a 'body wisdom desire' versus an emotional craving."[81]

Trap

Grocery shopping with family members.

This might seem like a good idea, but multiple opinions will lead to unnecessary purchases, and unnecessary purchases lead to temptation. If possible, make your list, check it twice, and stick with it. Alone.

Trick
When you're faced with a plateful of high-fat foods at a party or special event, tell yourself, "I'm only going to eat half of everything on my plate." Then take your time, making sure you chat with those nearby as you consume a smaller quantity than usual.

Testimony

When I got really sick a couple of years ago, all I wanted was to feel better. I wanted the pain to stop. So I chose healthy foods and did what my doctor recommended. I felt better after a short time and then really started doing well after about eight months. Then I started adding a few "no-no" foods. Just a little here, a little there, until I was eating more and more of them. Funny how a little leaven affects the whole lump. Those little bites grew like yeasty bread.

Deb Ullrick

Treasure

Blessed is the man who perseveres under trial,
because when he has stood the test,
he will receive the crown of life that
God has promised to those who love him.
James 1:12

Thought for the Day

From the time we were children, we pondered the word *forever*. It seemed like a mighty long time. Forever had no beginning and no end. Forever was an endless horizon, sweeping out with all its colors, holding us captive in our imaginations. And forever, at least for the health-conscious eater, can seem like a mighty long time. But when you come to understand that healthy eating isn't a punishment—it's a joy!—then, suddenly, forever just makes sense.

Turning Your Focus

Memorize a good, clean joke you can share
with your friends and loved ones.

Trusting God

Lord, I'm glad I don't have to dread the forevers associated with healthy eating. Please remind me that this is a joyful journey, not a never-ending diet. It is a lifestyle change that I can and should enjoy. Amen.

Today's Food Choices

(List all the foods you've eaten today)

_____

_____

_____

_____

Thoughts on Paper (Daily Journal Entry)

Feast on the Word

Tickler
*The journey of a thousand pounds
begins with a single burger.*
Chris O'Brien

Tidbit
Did You Know?

Some people eat when they're bored, simply because they can't think of anything better to do. Instead of reaching for a cookie or a snack cake, grab your Bible and head outside for some time alone with the Lord.

······· Trap ·······

Skipping meals will help me lose weight.

"If you stop eating regularly, your body will. . .hold on to its reserves. The body goes into 'starvation' mode, in. . .fear of not getting food soon. There is also the danger that by not eating all day you will overeat or binge in the evening."[82]

Trick
Drop one level of fat content in the milk you choose. For example, if you currently use 2 percent, switch to 1 percent. If you prefer whole milk, try 2 percent.[83]

Testimony

My dieting stories all seem to end with "emotional interruptions" that find me eating or snacking to relieve the "stress." *Boing* goes the diet—again. One thing that worked all the time, if I disciplined myself to do it, was reading my Bible. If I'd eaten a meal but went away still feeling hungry—particularly by mid-afternoon—I'd read my Bible and the hunger would always disappear. You know, the Bread of Life always fills you up!

Sue Timm

Treasure

*Let the word of Christ dwell in you richly
as you teach and admonish one another with all wisdom.*
COLOSSIANS 3:16

Thought for the Day

Who or what we turn to when we're hurting is very telling. If we turn to food, seeking an escape from the pain, we usually end up creating more pain. Instead, we need to turn to the Word of God on a daily basis, particularly if we are struggling. There we will find consolation, hope, strength, and joy. We can truly feast on the Word of God, devouring it like a healthy meal. We can then walk away from our "mealtimes" without the guilt, the despair, or the unwanted pounds.

Consider sponsoring a child in a foreign country.

Trusting God

Lord, thank You for giving us Your Word. It brings life and health to this body of mine and it energizes my soul, too. Thank You for sharing Your precepts and Your wisdom through the pages of the Bible. Remind me daily to stay close to You by getting into Your Word. Amen.

Today's Food Choices

(List all the foods you've eaten today)

_____

_____

_____

_____

Thoughts on Paper (Daily Journal Entry)

_____

_____

_____

_____

_____

_____

_____

Annie,
Stick to Your Guns

Tickler
To promise not to do a thing is
the surest way in the world to make
a body want to go and do that very thing.
Mark Twain, *The Adventures of Tom Sawyer*

Tidbit
Did You Know?

"It's not lack of willpower that causes us to give up dieting; it's lack of desire."[84]

⸱⸱⸱⸱⸱⸱⸱⸱⸱⸱⸱⸱⸱⸱⸱⸱⸱⸱⸱⸱⸱(Trap)⸱⸱⸱⸱⸱⸱⸱⸱⸱⸱⸱⸱⸱⸱⸱⸱

Party foods.

Just about the time you think you've got it made, you're invited to a party for a good friend. Finger foods abound, especially those little egg rolls you love so much and that fabulous cheese dip. Finger foods can be deceptive. They don't really fill you up, so you nibble more than you should, and they're loaded with calories and carbohydrates. Try eating a salad before going to a party. When you arrive, spend more time with your friend and less at the buffet table.

Trick

Be happy. Don't act as if resisting tempting foods is killing you.[85]

Testimony

It will be little by little and moment by moment, but I know with God's grace and His help I can do this. To learn that it isn't about weight loss and body size, but about obedience really helped me. At least for today, which is all I have anyway, right? I have no guarantee for tomorrow, only today. So today I will choose whom I will serve. . .and I choose the Lord.

Deb Ullrick

Treasure

I have fought the good fight,
I have finished the race,
I have kept the faith.
2 TIMOTHY 4:7

Thought for the Day

Sticking to your guns is possible—even in the midst of a party atmosphere. When you're faced with a table full of goodies with no nutritional content, reach for the vegetables and fruit first. Then, if you're truly hungry afterwards, take tiny portions of the things you love. Eat slowly as you make your rounds to visit friends. Don't make the evening about the food; make it about the people. There will always be parties. You will forever be faced with the temptation to do the wrong thing. A little nibbling won't hurt you, but filling your plate with nachos, smoked sausages, and cheese-cake might.

Turning Your Focus

Wave to a neighbor you've been at odds with (or barely know).

Trusting God

Sometimes, Lord, the goodies in my life aren't so good. Sometimes I don't stick to my guns and give in to temptation, only to face regret afterward. Help me to overcome temptation and to stand firm in my convictions. And help me to forgive myself when I stumble and fall. Amen.

Today's Food Choices

(List all the foods you've eaten today)

_____

_____

_____

_____

Thoughts on Paper (Daily Journal Entry)

_____

_____

_____

_____

_____

_____

_____

_____

_____

_____

_____

_____

_____

_____

_____

_____

_____

_____

_____

The "Happily Ever After" Mindset

Tickler

You have within you now all the elements that are necessary to make you all that the Father dreamed that you would be in Christ.
E. W. Kenyon

Tidbit
Did You Know?

"Ninety-five percent of all dieters will regain their lost weight in one to five years."[86]

· · · · · · · · · · · · · · (Trap) · · · · · · · · · · · · · · ·

Leading a sedentary lifestyle.

Since the invention of the television, we have become sedentary people. After sitting at a computer desk all day, we settle down on the sofa for an evening of rest and relaxation in front of the TV. Up and at 'em, folks. Time to replace sedentary with energetic.

Trick

Clean during commercials. Here's a trick I learned years ago. If you do sit to watch a TV show, make yourself get up during every commercial and clean something. In fact, go on a cleaning spree. Challenge yourself to see how much you can get done during one commercial. You'll be surprised at how much you accomplish, and you might actually forget you were watching television in the first place.

Treat

Low-fat hot cocoa. On those evenings when you must sit and rest, try a mug of low-fat hot cocoa. There are several brands and varieties available. You can even add a marshmallow or two. Just be careful not to overdo it.

Testimony

One thing I've learned is that I have a choice about what I'm putting into my body. Sometimes I make myself think, "Okay, what am I eating? Is this for fuel or for fat?" My body needs fuel to run, just like a car does. If I put junk in it, I'm still craving, and up goes the scale. But now I feel empowered with the knowledge that I can control what I eat. Self-control—what a great fruit of the Spirit. I might not have it all the time, but I'm getting there.

Lynette Sowell

Treasure

That is why I am suffering as I am.
Yet I am not ashamed,
because I know whom I have believed,
and am convinced that he is able to guard
what I have entrusted to him for that day.
2 TIMOTHY 1:12

Thought for the Day

The "happily ever after" mind-set. It's something we came to know as children reading fairy tales. In the end, the girl gets the handsome prince and they live happily ever after. There's no mention of a mortgage, electric bill, or car payment. In other words, no mention of stress. But in the real world, stress abounds and can cause us to lose focus. When you've made progress in both your thinking and your eating, it's easy to think you'll continue on without any interruptions to your overall plan for success. But sometimes life intervenes. Sometimes you're thrown off course. You will still make mistakes. Just don't be too hard on yourself.

-------------------------- (Turning Your Focus) --------------------------

Donate to a charity those clothes that no longer fit.

Trusting God

Lord, help me through the "not so pretty" times. Remind me of the progress I've made and encourage me to keep going, no matter what. And when I'm down, please remind me that sometimes the "frogs" of life turn out to be princes. Amen.

Today's Food Choices

(List all the foods you've eaten today)

_____

_____

_____

_____

Thoughts on Paper (Daily Journal Entry)

The Promised Land

Tickler
Rich, fatty foods are like destiny:
they, too, shape our ends.
Author Unknown

Tidbit
Did You Know?

Statistics show that up to one-third of deaths from cancer and heart disease could be prevented by healthier eating.[87]

Trap

One problem the Israelites had as they approached the Promised Land was their fear of crossing the Jordan River. God has brought you this far. Don't let your fear of the unknown stop you now. Cross on over.

Trick
Instead of having "cheat days" (such as splurging one day per week), consider smaller cheats, like eating a bite-sized candy bar or fat-free pudding several times a week. That way you won't feel so deprived.

Testimony

As I think of the most successful weight-loss program I've done, I remember that it wasn't intended to be a "weight-loss program" at all. About three years ago, our entire congregation went on a forty-day fast. I started out on liquids, then added vegetables, but no breads or sweets. By the end of the fast, I had lost about thirty pounds and had an I-can-do-all-things-through-Christ attitude. I've gained some of the weight back, but I never give up; I believe we can conquer the flesh. Since then, I've tried a lot of other programs, and I'm figuring out that diligence and moderation are what work. I'll keep trying.

Beth Ann Ziarnik

Treasure

*In their hunger you gave them bread from heaven
and in their thirst you brought them water from the rock;
you told them to go in and take possession of the land
you had sworn with uplifted hand to give them.*
NEHEMIAH 9:15

Thought for the Day

We've always equated the Promised Land with "arriving." It's the proverbial land of milk and honey. When we've reached the Promised Land, we tell ourselves, we can eat anything we want and remain slim and trim. After all, we've crossed the Red Sea with the enemy at our tail. We've marched through the desert, bravely facing the dangers. We've "done our time" at the bitter waters. And we've crossed the Jordan River, prepared for all of the delights of the Promised Land—only to discover that the "destination" isn't exactly what we thought it was. When a healthy eater "arrives" at his or her target weight, the journey has not ended. On the contrary, the Promised Land for the healthy eater is not a "place," it's a lifestyle.

······················ (Turning Your Focus) ··············

Pack a special note in your child's or spouse's lunch.

Trusting God

Oh Lord, I am so grateful. Grateful for Your grace and Your goodness. Grateful for Your wisdom and direction. Grateful for the changes I've seen in my life, which I know come as a result of following You. Thank You for leading me in Your ways. I give myself over to Your plan for my life, my health, and my future. Amen.

Today's Food Choices

(List all the foods you've eaten today)

_____

_____

_____

_____

Thoughts on Paper (Daily Journal Entry)

Renewed, All Things New

Tickler

You know you are dieting when postage stamps taste good.
Anonymous

Tidbit
Did You Know?

Most Americans (63 percent) are more concerned today than they were ten years ago about the healthfulness of the foods they eat. More than three-fourths (77 percent) say they are eating more healthfully, and almost 40 percent report exercising more than they did ten years ago.[88]

.... (Trap) ....

Thinking you've "arrived."

Even if you've reached your initial weight-loss goal, it's not time to settle back quite yet. Remember, the enemy would like to lure you into the trap of thinking the race is over.

Trick
"It's a good idea not to let yourself get too hungry before eating a meal or snack, because this is a surefire way to encourage overeating. Drinking sufficient water throughout the day (eight to ten glasses is generally recommended) will not only serve to keep you well hydrated, but will also help you feel less hungry."[89]

Testimony

If my heart doesn't change, it doesn't matter what I do to change the outside. Diet, exercise, or whatever, I won't be truly free from bondage until my heart is transformed. I need to let the Word of God transform me, and I need to desire obedience more than food. I haven't arrived yet, but then God isn't finished with me either. My heart still needs an overhaul job.

Deb Ullrick

Treasure

His master replied,
"Well done, good and faithful servant!
You have been faithful with a few things;
I will put you in charge of many things.
Come and share your master's happiness!"
MATTHEW 25:23

Thought for the Day

So here we are, arriving at the point where we thought the journey would end, only to discover that the race goes on forever. Why? It's simple: The Lord wants us to exercise diligence in our walk with Him. Just like reading the Word and praying, we need to care for our bodies day in and day out. We need to watch what we eat, and we need to get as much exercise as is reasonable. And we need to do something else, too. We need to stop worrying so much about what other people think about how we look. When we reach that point, we have truly progressed, whether we've lost two pounds or twenty-two. Congratulations on your progress! May God continue to bless you as you circle the track one more time.

························(Turning Your Focus)·············

Consider making a magazine subscription purchase
for a friend who might not be able to afford it.

Trusting God

Lord, I'm so grateful for all You've taught me in the past few months. I wholeheartedly give myself to You. I recognize that this body isn't mine; it's Yours. Thank You for entrusting it to me. I'm going to do my best to care for it as I continue on my journey toward good health. Amen.

Today's Food Choices

(List all the foods you've eaten today)

_____

_____

_____

_____

Thoughts on Paper (Daily Journal Entry)

He Must Increase

Congratulations, healthy eaters! Whether or not you've reached your target weight is irrelevant. You have run the race like a winner. You have progressed in your thinking and in your physical body. You now care as you have never cared before.

Doesn't it feel great to see lasting changes in your life? Doesn't it give you a sense of satisfaction to know that you've overcome addictions and developed new patterns? And aren't you glad you've had a chance to share a few laughs along the way? What better way to overcome obstacles than through the joy of the Lord, which brings strength.

As you look ahead to a healthy future, know that the Lord loves you. He loved you when you started this journey, and He loves you now. He loves you when you make right choices, and He loves you when you make mistakes. Nothing about His love for you has changed along the way. And He wants you to love yourself, as well—not in a prideful sort of way, but in a love-my-neighbor-as-myself sort of way.

There will be plenty of opportunities in the days ahead to make good choices. As you gear up to circle the track once again, take time to thank the Lord for what He's done in your life so far. He gives strength for the journey and encourages us in love. What an awesome God we serve! All the more reason He must increase in our lives. As we decrease, of course.

May God bless you on your journey.

He must increase,
but I must decrease.

John 3:30 NKJV

Endnotes

Facts footnoted in *I Must Decrease* were taken from reputable Web sites, at the following Web addresses, as of the time of this writing. Due to the ever-changing nature of the Internet, however, some facts quoted may no longer be available at these addresses.

1. http://www.horseracing.net/horseracingquotes.htm
2. http://www.niddk.nih.gov/publications/for_life.htm#your plan
3. http://www.national-raisin.com/raisins/health_benefits.html
4. http://womensissues.about.com/cs/bodyimage/a/bodyimagestats.htm
5. http://workplaceblues.com/health/statistics.asp
6. http://www.angelfire.com/blues/danthedietman
7. http://www.okweightloss.com/aboutobesity.phtml
8. http://www.niddk.nih.gov/health/nutrit/publications/understanding.htm
9. http://www.foodfunandfacts.com/foodtrivia.htm
10. http://www.isostar.com/public/content/exercise.htm
11. http://akak.essortment.com/healthbananas_rjyz.htm
12. http://womensissues.about.com/cs/bodyimage/a/bodyimagestats.htm
13. http://www.am-i-fat.com
14. http://www.angelfire.com/blues/danthedietman
15. http://www.betterhealth.vic.gov.au/bhcv2/bhcarticles.nsf/pages/Body_image_issues_for_women?OpenDocument
16. http://www.normaleating.com/fourstages.php
17. http://www.niddk.nih.gov/health/nutrit/pubs/wtloss/wtloss.htm#diet

18. http://www.whfoods.com/genpage.php?tname=foodspice&
    dbid=134

19. http://www.nhlbi.nih.gov/health/public/heart/obesity/lose_wt/
    recommen.htm

20. http://halife.com/family/food/asparagus.html

21. http://nutrition.about.com/library/weekly/aa030701a.htm; See
    also www.caloriecontrol.org/pr070303.html.

22. http://www.emptytomb.org/lifestylestat.html

23. http://www.cdc.gov/nchs/releases/03news/physicalactivity.htm

24. http://www.cancer.org/docroot/PED/content/PED_3_1x_
    Body_Mass_Index_Calculator.asp

25. http://workplaceblues.com/eating/20ways.asp

26. http://agnews.tamu.edu/dailynews/stories/HORT/Jun1902a.htm

27. http://www.medhelp.org/NIHlib/GF-367.html

28. http://www.niddk.nih.gov/publications/understanding.
    htm#Psychological

29. http://www.healthywithin.com/stats.htm

30. http://www.wholehealthmd.com/hc/depression/chronic_
    dietaryadvice/1,1718,453,00.html

31. http://www.appleproducts.org/research.html

32. http://www.uic.edu/orgs/sci-adapt/salt.html

33. http://www.gourmetgarlicgardens.com/health.htm

34. http://nutrition.about.com/library/weekly/aa022303a.htm

35. http://www.angelfire.com/blues/danthedietman

36. http://www.cdc.gov/nchs/releases/03news/physicalactivity.
    htm

37. http://www.adagio.com/info/health_benefits/news_4.html?SID
    =710a97d81d432c939bc35956b66a61f1

38. http://www.cdc.gov/nccdphp/sgr/ataglan.htm

39. http://www.studenthealth.co.uk/leaflets/DietTricks&Tips.htm

40. http://www.michigan.gov/mda/0,1607,7-125-1570_2468_
    2471-38102— ,00.html

41. http://weightloss-and-diet-facts.com/more-dieting-failures.htm

42. http://www.childstats.gov/ac1999/heirel.asp;
www.childstats.gov/ac2004/tables/econ4b.asp

43. http://www.anred.com/who.html

44. http://www.campusblues.com/body_image1_1.asp

45. http://www.emptytomb.org/lifestylestat.html

46. http://www.olen.com/food/book.html

47. http://www.practicalweightloss.com/nutrition/articles/lose-fat/
lose-weight-without-being-hungry.html

48. http://www.cdc.gov/nccdphp/sgr/ataglan.htm

49. http://www.healthy-dining.com/facts.htm

50. http://www.olen.com/food/book.html

51. http://www.foodfunandfacts.com/foodtrivia.htm

52. http://nutrition.about.com/library/weekly/aa092700a.htm

53. http://www.nswcc.org.au/editorial.asp?pageid=363

54. http://content.health.msn.com/content/article/79/96309.htm

55. http://www.campusblues.com/body_image1_1.asp

56. http://www.cbsnews.com/stories/2003/06/23/earlyshow/
health/health_news/main559830.shtml

57. http://library.adoption.com/Nutrition-Diet-Food/in-Dieting/
article/3050/1.html

58. http://www.nutritionexplorations.org/parents/snack-smart.asp

59. http://www.emptytomb.org/lifestylestat.html

60. http://nutrition.about.com/library/weekly/aa070202a.htm

61. http://nutrition.about.com/library/weekly/aa081500a.htm

62. http://www.girlpower.gov/girlarea/bodywise/eatingdisorders/
statistics.htm

63. http://www.anred.com/stats.html

64. http://www.emptytomb.org/lifestylestat.html

65. http://nutrition.about.com/library/weekly/aa112202a.htm

66. http://womensissues.about.com/cs/bodyimage/a/bodyimages-

tats.htm

67. http://www.exercare.com/results/thepulse/Issue3-Apr2004.htm

68. http://www.dietbites.com/article0098.html

69. http://www.hardthinkers.com/mt/archives/000039.html

70. http://www.valleyfig.com/c_figs/index.htm

71. http://www.holistic-online.com/Humor_Therapy/humor_therapy_benefits.htm

72. http://www.herhealthandbeauty.com/articles/body_acceptance.htm

73. http://health.discovery.com/centers/weightloss/articles/pennplan/tips.html

74. http://www.healthywithin.com/stats.htm

75. http://www.groundworkgreaternottingham.org.uk/fig/healthy

76. http://www.skyhighway.com/~turtleway/Articles/yoyoemo.html

77. http://www.unitedwaytwincities.org/news/tipsheets/hl_nutrition.cfm

78. http://my.webmd.com/content/article/85/98822.htm

79. http://www.practicalweightloss.com/nutrition/articles/lose-fat/lose-weight-without-being-hungry.html

80. http://www.campusblues.com/body_image1_1.asp

81. http://www.normaleating.com/fourstages.php

82. http://www.weightlossresources.co.uk/login/news_features/diet_facts.htm

83. http://www.praize.com/health/weightloss.html

84. http://www.annecollins.com/weight_loss_tips/willpower.htm

85. http://www.weightremedy.net/dietingtips.html

86. http://www.healthywithin.com/stats.htm

87. http://www.groundworkgreaternottingham.org.uk/fig/healthy

88. http://www.healthy-dining.com/facts.htm

89. http://www.mamashealth.com/hmeals/snack.asp

Notes

Notes

Notes

Notes

_____

_____

_____

_____

_____

_____

_____

_____

_____

_____

_____

_____

_____

_____

_____

_____

_____

Notes

Notes

Notes

Notes

Notes

Other Books from
Barbour Publishing

The Neurotic's Guide to God and Love
by Lance Moore
Does Murphy's Law feel like your personal
motto? With warmth and humor, *The Neurotic's
Guide. . .* identifies the common mistakes that
prevent Christians from living abundantly.
192 pages / $8.97
ISBN 1-59310-972-5

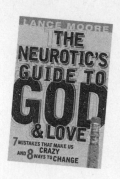

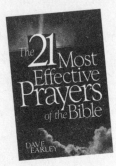

The 21 Most Effective Prayers of the Bible
by Dave Earley
Want to know how to pray? Use the Word
of God as your guide! This easy-to-read
volume studies twenty-one heartfelt prayers
from the Bible that produced results.
176 pages / $7.97
ISBN 1-59310-605-X

Another Fine Mess, Lord!
by Karon Phillips Goodman
It's time to get more out of life! In the every-
day stress and frustration, you can find God's
abundance in simplicity, order, and insight.
192 pages / $7.97
ISBN 1-59310-606-8

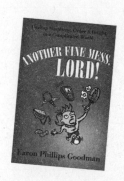

Available wherever Christian books are sold.